THE KETO COACH:
How to Lose Fat and Get Healthy Without Medicine

John Hutmacher

2021

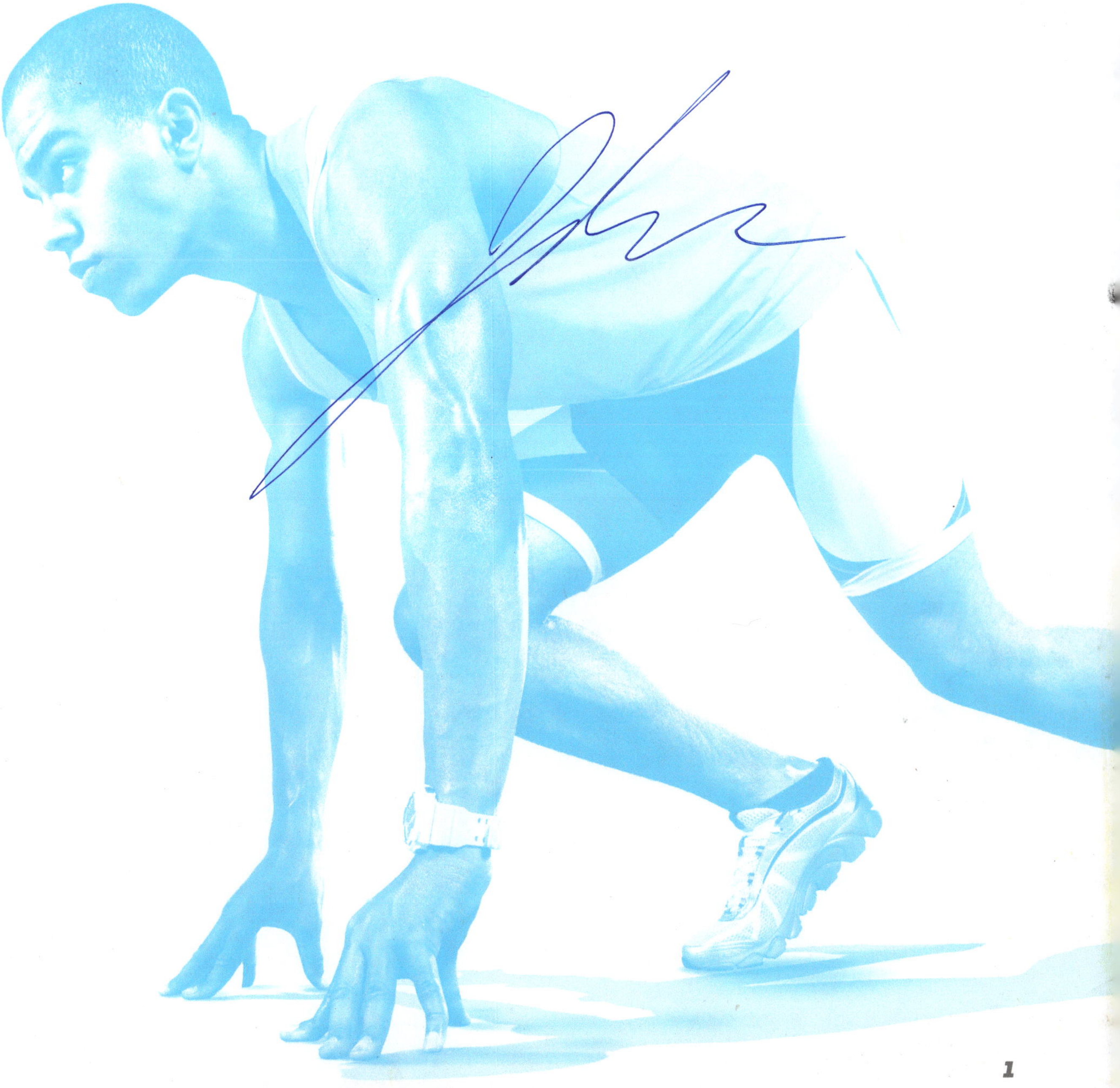

CONTENTS

INTRODUCTION

THE KETO COACH

We didn't start fat, but look at us now. How did this happen? I won "Best Body" in high school, and here I am in November 2016 (bottom left). Six months later I took the second picture.

Like many of you, I've struggled since high school to keep the weight off. Especially after the birth of my first child, I had a really hard time. Starting when I was around twenty-nine, my exercise routine dropped off, I began eating whatever was around the house, and my lifestyle became very sedentary.

For my entire thirties, my weight bounced between 210 and 230 pounds, with 230 being the high point. I would make attempts to get back into shape and drop the pounds. Just like all of us, I knew the classical weight loss formula: working out more and eating less.

I would get up at 4:30 a.m. and lift weights and walk for an hour. I would restrict my diet to a thousand calories a day. I have always had a lot of discipline, and I worked very hard at getting my body back to what it had been. The problem was, I wasn't losing any weight.

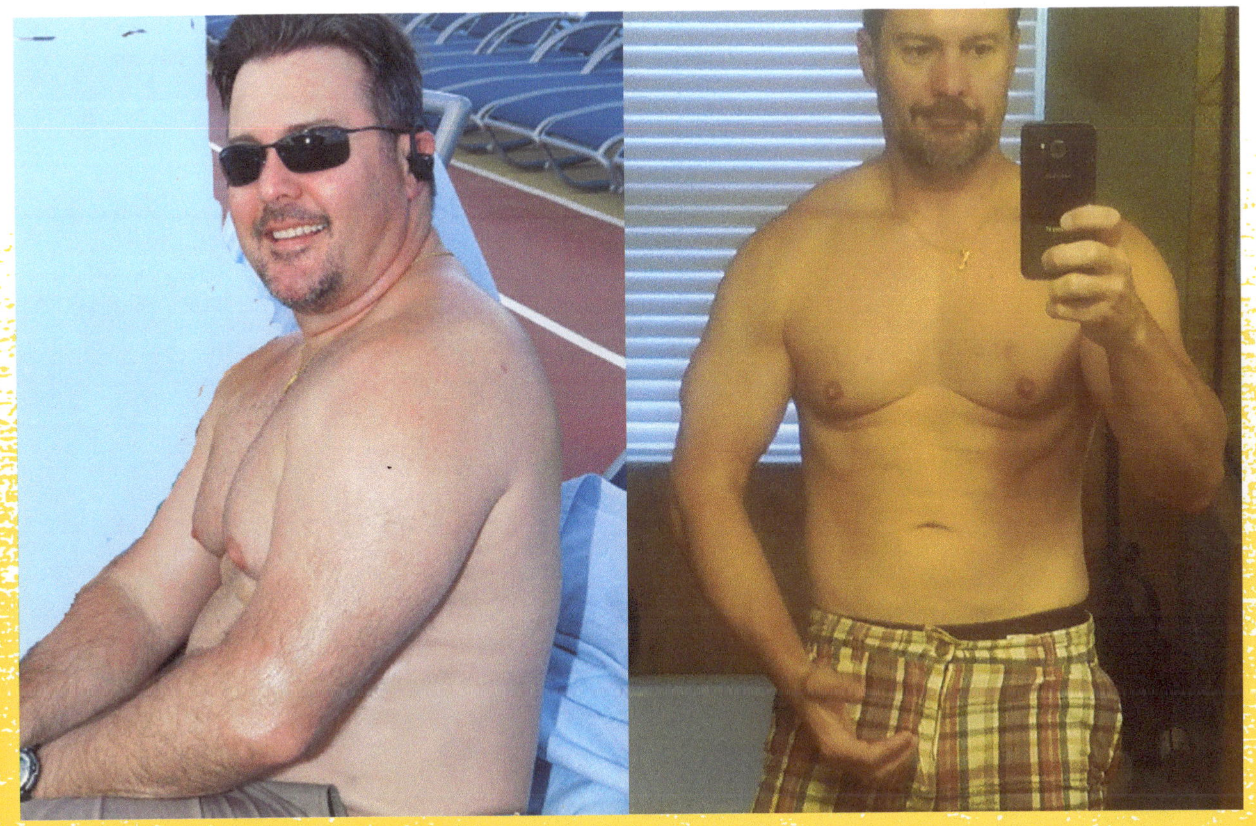

THIS IS THE BOOK THAT BREAKS IT ALL DOWN FOR YOU. YOU CAN READ KETO COACH IN ONE SITTING AND HAVE ALL THE TOOLS TO GET STARTED ON YOUR OWN KETO JOURNEY.

Was I destined to be fat forever?

One day I was walking on the treadmill (per usual) watching CNBC. An interview came on with entrepreneur and author, Tim Ferriss. Most of the interview was about his business strategies, but I was fascinated by the lifestyle stuff he kept talking about; intermittent fasting, burning calories from the fat your body already has—totally new ways of thinking about how our body uses and stores energy.

I immediately bought Ferriss's book, *Tools of Titans*, where—among many other topics—he talked about fasting as a way to heal the body.[1] He described what he learned from nutrition expert, Doctor Dom (Dr. Dominic D'Agostino): on a three-day fast you eventually enter a metabolic state or "fat burning mode" called **ketosis**. You lose weight not because of calorie restriction, but because of this different metabolic state you have triggered in your body.

He explained that we have two metabolic states: **sugar** burning mode and **fat** burning mode. Because of our modern diet, most of us exist in sugar burning mode. But, after just two days of not eating, you switch fuel sources and start burning fat instead.

So did you just have to not eat forever? How was this different than starving yourself? The next part blew my mind. *Dr. Dom had a way to stay in fat burning mode once he started eating again.* If we continue eating a certain way, we can stay in this fat burning mode, known as ketosis, indefinitely.

"*What?*" I thought.

I had to know more, so I jumped on the web and found my way to www.dietdoctor.com where I learned as much as I could about the Ketogenic Diet. I bought the necessary materials and began my own keto journey.

That was February 2017. When, I started on this new diet, or really, this new lifestyle, I weighed 220 pounds.

Six months later, I was in the best shape of my life. Truly. I was 16% body fat, a number I hadn't been close to in years. My weight still fluctuated, but at its lowest I was at 173 pounds, just two pounds more than my high school senior year wrestling weight of 171 pounds. I was back to a 28-inch waistline.

But that doesn't begin to tell the whole story. Eating a keto diet isn't just about losing weight, it's about improving your health overall.

If you want to:

* Understand how the interaction of hormones in your body affects your weight
* Increase energy levels
* Reduce brain fog
* Combat autoimmune diseases without relying so heavily on medicine
* Reduce overall inflammation
* Understand the unique needs of your body—how it refuels, how it stores energy, and how to give it what it wants

1 Ferriss, Tim. *Tools of Titans*. Houghton Mifflin Harcourt, New York, 2016.

* How to find balance in your life and enjoy food with feast and fast

And go beyond simple ketosis by:

* Eating a plant-based diet that avoids foods that increase inflammation
* Use intermittent fasting as a powerful tool to reset your body
* Build muscle and fitness without spending your life in the gym

... then this book is for you.

When I began eating a keto diet, there wasn't much information out there. I found the initial guides good, but unsatisfying. I wanted to understand not just what I was eating but why: how it worked and all the science behind it.

So, I spent hours reading books, tracking down studies, and watching endless hours of YouTube videos of doctors, scientists, and dieticians discussing ketosis. I synthesized everything I learned and implemented my take on the keto diet. Even after my initial positive results, I continued to be curious about how to refine my process. I became my own guinea pig.

All the supplements, blood test kits, and two-week plans? I've tried them. I have used every blood meter, lengthened my fasting to more than a week, gone on cruises and stuffed my face and then experimented with how quickly the weight comes off when I go back on my diet. The stuff that worked went in a Word document called "Coaching." The document quickly became a sprawling mess as I delved deeper and deeper into the nuances of ketosis. In addition, I had extra pages of detailed notes and years of spreadsheets tracking my own daily body stats.

When people saw the results I had achieved, they became curious about the ketogenic diet. This "Coaching" document was what I sent them to help get them started. While there were plenty of existing excellent resources to share with them, most people wouldn't get past the introductions of my favorite books. They just wanted the nitty-gritty: what is ketosis, how does it work, and how do I get going?

You've heard all the hype about ketosis. Maybe you've even done a little research but immediately got overwhelmed by the amount of information out there. It's hard to tell what's real, what's useful, and how deep you need to go.

There's enough science in here so you know why the diet is working, but not so much that you need to read around it in order to effectively implement the diet.

Later chapters in the book will address more advanced topics: for example, how to manage ketosis for bodybuilding or how female hormones influence weight loss cycles, even in ketosis. Most importantly, I will introduce in-depth intermittent fasting, one of the most powerful tools in my nutritional toolkit. Finally, in the back of the book, you will find reference guides for grocery shopping, recipes, workouts, and more.

Every day I meet people who aren't living the life they want because of the extra weight they are carrying as well as the diseases and conditions they have been diagnosed with that are caused by our modern diet. I was there with you: pre-diabetic, with no energy to play with my children or get out and enjoy life. Constantly trying different diets and workout routines with no real progress being made. But, with the powerful tools contained in this book, I know you will have results. You will have more energy and be enjoying life more fully soon. Jump in with me and give it a try.

CHAPTER 1: INTRODUCTION TO KETOSIS

THE WRONG INFORMATION

We've been told our entire lives that calories in and calories out plus moving more equals weight loss.

Here's the thing: it's total crap.

There is no science backing up this formula, and yet it has been popular for more than fifty years.

The second law of thermodynamics says that energy is conserved. This is known as energy balance and is where the basic idea of calories in and calories out comes from. If you apply this thinking to your body, then calorie restriction becomes a viable and practical way to lose weight.

But what's true in the universe isn't true in the human body. For starters, energy balance way oversimplifies how our bodies work, pretending there is only one variable that affects how we use and store energy. Study after study show that this methodology is wrong.[2]

Under a Standard American Diet (SAD), if you reduce your calorie intake below the BMR (Basal Metabolic Rate), your body will slow its metabolism to match the lower calorie intake. You might—*might*—lose some weight initially, but most likely that will drop off pretty quickly. Then when you get frustrated that your weight loss has stopped and you go back to eating regular-sized meals, your body isn't accustomed to the "excess" calories you used to eat without experiencing weight gain. And you gain weight at a calorie intake that would have maintained your weight before.

That's the real kicker: just restricting your calories will most likely lead to you gaining more weight.

The problem is that we treat all calories as equal. Not true.

There are actually **three sources** of calories: **carbohydrates, proteins, and fats.** The body processes and also stores these calorie sources differently. In "calories in and calories out," the model assumes only one storage tank that we fill and withdraw from. This is also wrong. In addition to the three different ways we can fill our storage tanks via the different caloric sources, we have **two** actual storage tanks: **glycogen and fat.** *[FIG 1.1]*

2 https://www.dovepress.com/the-western-diet-and-lifestyle-and-diseases-of-civilization-peer-reviewed-article-RRCC

The body runs on glucose, or blood sugar, the common energy currency. Our cells only need so much energy at a time, so excess glucose is pushed out of the blood and stored first as glycogen. Glycogen is stored in modest amounts in the skeletal muscle and liver, roughly 400 and 500 grams, respectively. A gram of carbohydrate is about 4 kilocalories (kcals), so you can store about 1,600 to 2,000 kcals in your carbohydrate, or glycogen, fuel tank. Think of this as the short-term fuel tank. After this is full, your body moves on to the second fuel tank, the fat fuel tank.

In the fat fuel tank, the body stores fatty acids in the form of triglycerides, three fatty acids linked by a single three-carbon glycerol molecule. Unlike the limited storage of glycogen, there is no limit on fat storage. *[FIG 1.2]*

Fat is denser than glucose, providing 9 kcals per gram. Even a very lean person, someone with, let's say, 10 % body fat and 150 pounds, still has 15 pounds of fat, or over 45,000 stored calories. This is more than 30 times the energy that exists in our stored sugar fuel tank. Most of us carry around much more fat than that.

I was at almost 30% body fat when I started my journey.

Here is the math on my body, pre-keto:

230 pounds x 30% body fat
*= **69 pounds of fat***

*69 pounds of fat x 3,500 calories per pound = **241,500 stored calories***

FIG 1.1 ***THOMAS DELAUER'S – KETOX PROGRAM***

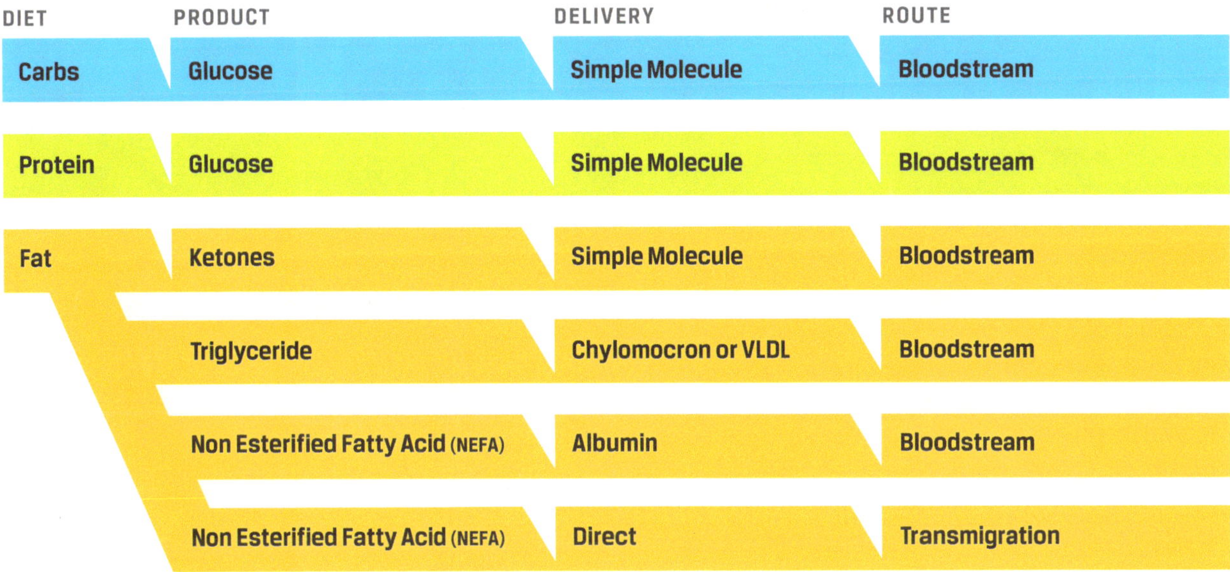

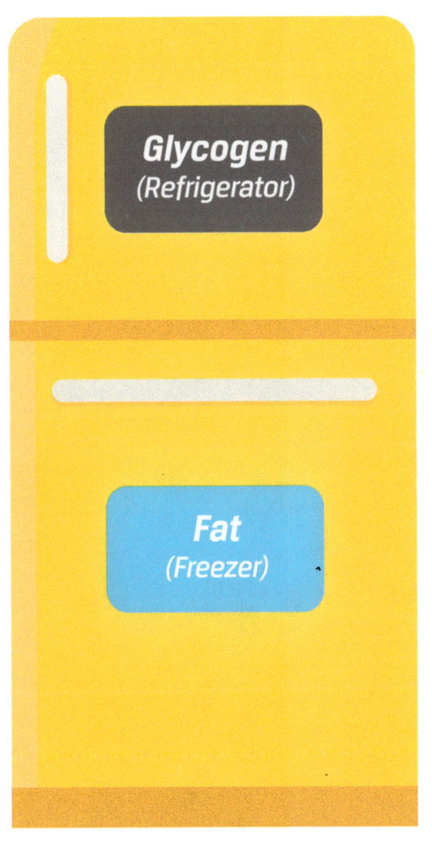

FIG 1.2 ***Glycogen / Fat Storage***

Considering an average workout burns less than 300 calories, those 241,500 calories were more than enough to last me a very long time.

Excess amounts of the three energy sources are processed differently in the body. Excess fat in the diet that is not burned will get placed into the fat storage tank, just like excess carbohydrates. Excess protein, on the other hand, is not stored directly. What is not used gets converted by the liver into glucose for storage.

So, How Do We Get Fat?

The answer lies not in counting calories but in our *hormones. The hormones floating around in the body tell the cells what to do with the calories we are taking in.* One hormone tells the body to store fat, and the other tells the body to release fat. It is crazy to me that when we discuss weight loss or health in general, we are so fixated on calories without looking at what is actually happening in our bodies.

I have explained what the sources of energy are and where energy is stored. But what is the process by which energy sources are converted into energy? What governs that? How does the body know what becomes glucose and what becomes fat? How does it know which tank to draw from?

All these processes are regulated by our body's hormones.

Understanding this interaction is where the answer lies in figuring out when we gain, lose, or retain weight.

What Is Fat?

So first let's understand that the terms "overweight" and "obese" just mean an over-accumulation of fat in your body.

But why does our body allow fat to accumulate?

Hormones

Insulin is the culprit. Simple. Insulin is the hormone that partitions energy in the blood to be stored. Are we going to use the short-term energy in our glycogen tank, or are we going to use the long-term energy stored in our fat? Insulin directs this response.

Let's talk about insulin and hormone response.

According to an article in *SF Gate*, a normal fasting glucose level is 60 to 100 milligrams per deciliter. These levels shouldn't go over 200 mg/dl one hour after eating and 140 mg/dl two hours after eating. Most non-diabetics have below 120 mg/dl after two hours.[3] (This data will be especially useful once you get into measuring key indicators in your blood.)

Let's examine a key study of 50,000 women done by the NIH (National Institutes of Health) in the early 90's.[4] Twenty thousand of the women were chosen at random and were put on a low-fat diet with a 360-calorie restriction per day from their normal eating habits. The goal of the study was to understand whether low-fat diets prevent heart disease or cancer when put in practice.

The results were interesting. After eight years, the women in the study had only lost two pounds, even though their caloric intake was restricted by 20%. In addition, their waist circumference had actually *increased*. Why? They had lost lean muscle mass and gained fat.

If you just did the math on what they should have lost based on calories in versus calories out, they should have been losing 3 pounds a month—or 36 pounds per year—of fat. This is not what happened. In addition, and even worse, this low-fat diet was not shown to reduce heart disease or cancer.

One of the most popular versions of the low-fat diet is the *Biggest Loser* diet, the NBC show that ran from 2004-2016. On the show, under the advice of trainers, contestants cut their diets by 600 calories a day and exercise a lot. This is a popular implementation of the "move more, eat less" philosophy.

During the course of filming, the average contestant loses more than 100 pounds over three months—an amazing weight loss. They show contestants stepping on the scale during their final weigh-in with a totally changed physique.

What they never show is that almost all of the contestants regain the weight.

The actual stats done on one season of the show indicate that thirteen out of fourteen contestants regained all the weight they had lost, even though

ONE OF THE MOST POPULAR VERSIONS OF THE LOW-FAT DIET IS THE BIGGEST LOSER DIET, THE NBC SHOW...

This is a popular implementation of the "move more, eat less" philosophy...

What they never show is that almost all of the contestants regain the weight.

3 https://healthyeating.sfgate.com/high-sugar-level-after-meal-4348.html

4 "News from the Women's Health Initiative: Reducing Total Fat Intake May Have Small Effect on Risk of Breast Cancer, No Effect on Risk of Colorectal Cancer, Heart Disease, or Stroke," National Institutes of Health, February 7, 2006, https://www.nih.gov/news-events/news-releases/news-womens-health-initiative-reducing-total-fat-intake-may-have-small-effect-risk-breast-cancer-no-effect-risk-colorectal-cancer-heart-disease-or-stroke.

they continued eating less even after filming had ended.[5] The only one who didn't regain the weight had gastric bypass surgery to restrict their stomach capacity.

The reason these people all failed to keep the weight off is that the body will reduce metabolism to the total of calories coming in. Since their bodies weren't getting the same calories as before, their bodies slowed down their metabolism to match the calories coming in. So even on a lower diet of say, 2,000 calories, their body was now used to only 1,500 calories, leaving 500 to be stored.

So why does our metabolism react this way?

Insulin-Resistant Cells

Every time we eat, an insulin response is triggered. Once our insulin is too high, the body starts resisting it, requiring it to produce more insulin to push the glucose out of the bloodstream into the cells. This is where the real problem occurs. Insulin never comes back down to a level that will allow us to move into fat retrieval mode. Let me explain.

What happens is that insulin tells the body that there is too much blood sugar (glucose) in the blood stream to be used as energy and triggers the LPL receptor on the cell to store the glucose into the fat cells and muscle tissue for use later.

So how much glucose can the body use? Your blood normally only has about 5 grams of sugar in it. But the average person consumes *300 to 400 grams* of carbohydrates (glucose) in a day.

This means that much of what we eat during the day can't be used by the body at that moment in time. Blood sugar spikes. To fix this the body releases insulin to trigger the cells to remove the blood sugar and store it for later. Since we eat like this all the time, the body is in a constant state of trying to lower the blood sugar back down to normal levels.

With high levels of insulin present in the blood all the time, the cells start to ignore the insulin, or resist. This leads the body to become what is known as "insulin resistant." Since the body's blood sugar is still too high, the body produces even more insulin to get the cells to respond and remove and store the excess blood sugar. At some point the body cannot produce enough insulin to regulate the blood sugar. This is known as "Type 2 Diabetes."[6]

But Type 2 diabetes is not the only medical condition to result. In fact, a whole host of medical problems stems from insulin resistance. Metabolic syndrome, high blood pressure, high cholesterol, belly fat, fatty liver, diabetes, heart problems, inflammation, brain problems like Alzheimer's and dementia, decreased testosterone, cancer, and more (I explore Metabolic Syndrome in depth below).[7]

And yet we treat all of these diseases with separate drugs. Why?

Metabolic Syndrome

Metabolic Syndrome as described by the Mayo Clinic is a cluster of conditions that increase your risk of heart disease, stroke and diabetes:[8]

* Increased blood pressure
* High blood sugar
* Excess body fat around the waist
* Abnormal cholesterol or triglyceride levels

Three common measurements that indicate metabolic syndrome are:

* Fasting glucose over 100 mg/dl
* HDL level below 40 in men and 50 in women
* Triglycerides levels above 130mg/dl blood pressure top number over 138 and bottom number over 86[9]

To fix these numbers, we need to lower our insulin levels. To lower our insulin levels, we need to lower the sugar in our blood. To lower the sugar in our blood, we need to consume less sugar. To consume lower sugar, we need to limit our intake of carbohydrates in all forms. (You will get the game plan for this in Keto Diet Notes.)

What caused our body to work this way, only using a limited amount of energy at a time and putting the rest into long-term storage?

For over 2 million years, humans ate a hunter-gatherer's diet consisting mostly of animals and then some fruits and vegetable when they were found. Primitive humans operated in a feast-and-fast environment where food was scarce most of the time, thereby naturally restricting their calories. It has only been in the last hundred generations that we started farming our food and moved into cities. Our bodies have not had time to evolve to our new diet, especially in the United States, where our food culture is post-industrial.

Our bodies are always expecting famine, but we live in "feast" mode, constantly storing calories away to use later. We blast ourselves with sugar via our carb-heavy diet, so our glycogen tanks never empty. We never burn fat because we never need to.

5 Fothergill, Erin et al, Persistent metabolic adaptation 6 years after "The Biggest Loser" competition, Wiley Online Library, May 2, 2016, https://onlinelibrary.wiley.com/doi/abs/10.1002/oby.21538.

6 http://www.diabetes.org/diabetes-basics/type-2/

7 https://www.youtube.com/watch?v=tRPqYqa3oLA&feature=youtu.be

8 https://www.mayoclinic.org/diseases-conditions/metabolic-syndrome/symptoms-causes/syc-20351916

9 https://www.urmc.rochester.edu/encyclopedia/content.aspx?contenttypeid=85&contentid=P08342

Next we try to lose weight by restricting calories, but since our bodies are still in glucose-burning mode, we can't access our fat stores. Our body needs to be retrained to know how. So, without the ability to burn fat, our body goes into starvation mode. Those fat stores become even more precious—and untouchable. *[See "Recent Example" below.]*

Other Hormones

But understanding what is happening with your weight, energy levels, or general health isn't as simple as just focusing on insulin. While this is the key culprit, we have other hormones in our body that have a fundamental effect on our quality of life.

As the book progresses, we will learn more about the specific ways in which these hormones affect our keto journey (for example, most women will not experience linear weight loss while eating a ketogenic diet because of their sex hormones; see more in chapter 5).

For now, here is a brief introduction to the hormones that come into play.

THYROID HORMONE

People with low thyroid can have symptoms like dry skin, fatigue, cold intolerance, constipation, and weight gain. The thyroid hormone controls metabolism, so a high level of thyroid hormones results in you having a high metabolism, while a low-level thyroid hormone leads to a low metabolism. Your metabolism dictates whether you will burn 1,500 calories a day or 2,500, just at your resting rate. Weight gain is usually caused by a lower metabolism. This can be easily tested in your blood by your doctor.

You can increase your thyroid levels naturally by consuming adequate iodine. You can get iodine in fish, shellfish, kelp, and sea salt. I prefer a daily kelp supplement in a pill. This kelp supplement has natural iodine that will help increase thyroid

A Recent Example of the Effect of a Change in Diet:

Today the Pima have the highest incidence of obesity and diabetes in the Americas.[†] *The Pima used to be slender, physically active farmers and hunters. They are now sedentary wage earners, like the rest of Americans. It's easy to fall into the trap of believing that they are now obese because they don't move enough anymore, but the problem showed up much earlier—before the 1900s, even.*

In the early 1800s, there were reports of explorers' encounters with the Pima Indians. They were observed as being thin and very healthy. They raised crops and lived off the animals in the area. When the gold rush hit in 1846, the US government asked the Pima to feed people who were traveling west.

By the 1870s, the white settlers built a town, diverted the river used to irrigate the Pima's land, and hunted all the wildlife out of the area. Due to a shortage of food, the government stepped in with government rations to help the Pima. These rations consisted of white flour, coffee, and sugar.

This was when the Pima started getting obese, having diabetes, and being malnourished: all these health issues despite the fact that they were still in the fields working hard. They were still calorie-restricted. And yet, they were obese. What changed? The introduction of the flour and sugar.

† https://care.diabetesjournals.org/content/16/1/369

function. Also, get rid of GMO foods and veggies in your diet that have been sprayed with Round Up. Plant Paradox 7 disrupters (more on this later in chapter 4) will fix thyroid function.

SEX HORMONES

Sex hormones also affect your weight. PCOS is an endocrine disorder that elevates testosterone and insulin levels in women. Also, during menopause, women's estrogen drops and causes some weight gain (I have devoted an entire chapter to this; see more in chapter 5). For men, testosterone gradually declines over time. This can lead to slight weight gain.

STRESS HORMONES

Stress shows up as cortisol in the body. Cortisol increases hunger, which causes weight gain. Lack of sleep is the most common cause of elevated cortisol.[10] Exercise and more sleep will help counter this hormone that is working against your weight loss goals. Women are biologically more sensitive to cortisol, but increased cortisol affects both sexes. See specific tips for cortisol reduction in chapter 5.

How to Reverse Insulin Resistance Quickly

So, if restricting your calorie intake doesn't work to lose weight, what does? Remember how we have those two fuel sources: glucose (sugar and carbohydrates) and ketones (fat). So now we finally get to:

KETOSIS

Ketosis is a natural metabolic state where the body burns stored body fat to produce energy to live on. The liver converts fat to ketone bodies. Ketones are similar to the glucose energy molecule (blood sugar). But studies have shown the brain actually functions better on ketones than glucose.[11]

To get into ketosis, we first have to deplete our glycogen stores. This process won't happen overnight, especially if we are continuing to eat anything that refills them, including carbs and excess proteins. In fact, it can take between 48 hours to one week depending on carbohydrate intake and overall calorie intake.

GLYCOGEN STORES

Your body has between 400 to 500 grams of glycogen, which translates to 1,600–2,000 calories stored in muscles and liver. This is stored sugar; you must deplete this before the body will switch to burning fat for energy.

To do this, we need to remove the carbohydrates from our diet and keep our protein intake below 150 grams per day to keep the glycogen from being replenished. Once our blood sugar or glucose starts dropping from the lack of new glucose from food, the body will stop producing insulin to store away the excess blood sugar.

Now that insulin is low, the body will release the alternate hormone glucacon which will allow you to access your stored fat. Your liver will then start producing ketones from the fat you eat and your body fat. Ketones are an alternative source of energy for the body. Once your blood level of ketones are above 0.5 mmol/dL, this is known as ketosis.

(For faster results and reducing insulin, see chapter 3 on intermittent fasting.)

Keto Myths

Keto is a hot topic right now, but it isn't well understood. For example, training your body to burn fat by balancing your hormonal interactions probably isn't the first thing you think of when I mention keto.

Here are some of the other common misconceptions

* Am I going to lose muscle?
* Is my cholesterol going to go crazy?
* Will I have to eat keto forever?
* Is keto a fully protein diet?
* Why can't I just exercise to my goal weight and eat what I want?

Exercise is another arena in which popular myth exceeds scientific knowledge. We have many ideas about how to exercise that are totally ingrained in us that have no basis in scientific fact. For example, high-intensity cardio workouts that are an hour or more long can actually promote weight gain, especially in women. This book will recommend what kind of exercise to work into your lifestyle, but you will be surprised by how little is necessary to lose weight and maintain a healthy lifestyle

Please reference:
https://www.youtube.com/watch?v=-koeqbTufBO

10 https://www.health.harvard.edu/staying-healthy/why-stress-causes-people-to-overeat

11 https://blogs.scientificamerican.com/mind-guest-blog/the-fat-fueled-brain-unnatural-or-advantageous/

Myth #1 - You Need Carbs to Live [Gluconeogenesis]

Your body knows it can't always count on receiving three carb-based meals per day (our ancestors never ate that way), so it evolved a mechanism to make glucose out of different substances, such as lactate and amino acids. This process is called *gluconeogenesis*, and despite it being crucial to your survival, it is highly misunderstood. The clue to what this actually is, is in the name, *gluco*, meaning glucose; *neo*, meaning new; and *genesis*, meaning origin or creation. In summary, your cells use gluconeogenesis to ensure you don't die when there are no carbs in your system.

Our body uses gluconeogenesis to ensure you don't die when in ketosis. Just as too much glucose is toxic, too little can kill you, too. The brain also needs a little bit of glucose to work optimally, but not *only* glucose. Ketones can cover up to 70% of what your brain needs to work optimally, but not everything. This happens naturally after a meal, while you sleep, during a fast, and during an extended fast. Your total glucose goes down only because glycogenolysis, the breakdown of glycogen, declines as glycogen stores run out, but GNG stays the same. Note: *when your body runs out of glycogen, it relies completely on gluconeogenesis*. Researchers found that on keto, excess glucose made from gluconeogenesis was stored as glycogen instead of being used as fuel.[12]

Myth #2 - Calories Don't Matter

A lot of keto dieters think that you can eat as much as you want when in ketosis, and while not all calories are created equal (explained below), being in a caloric surplus day over day won't result in weight loss. Oh boy.

The first law of thermodynamics (or the law of conservation of energy) states that energy cannot be created or destroyed. When applied to weight control, this law translates to the basic formula: weight gain = energy (calories) in - energy (calories) out. This traditional viewpoint argues that the food eaten is unimportant and that a calorie is a calorie; to lose weight, create a calorie deficit by either eating less or burning more; to gain weight, increase caloric intake.

The loss of energy as heat through the thermic effect of food is consistent with the second law of thermodynamics, which states that some energy is always lost in any chemical reaction. The thermic effect of the different macronutrients varies, 2% of the energy for fat, and 25% of the energy for protein. Sources vary on the exact numbers, but nutrients from protein require much more energy to metabolize than fat and carbs. If you go with a thermic effect of 25% for protein and 2% for fat, this would mean that 100 calories of protein would end up as 75 calories, while 100 calories of fat would end up as 98 calories. Make sense?[13]

Myth #3 - Keto is Dangerous [Ketosis vs Ketoacidosis]

Many people confuse ketosis with ketoacidosis. Ketoacidosis, also known as diabetic ketoacidosis (DKA), is a potentially deadly situation when the body doesn't produce enough insulin, allowing you to have both high ketones and blood sugar at the same time. This is usually only a problem for type 1 diabetics who don't produce adequate levels of insulin to control blood sugar. Ketosis is when the body produces ketones by breaking down fat to make up for low glucose levels as fuel. In non-diabetics, blood sugar goes down and ketones come up, never getting close to ketoacidosis. The body regulates the production of ketones with the release of insulin, keeping the ketone levels in the blood well below ketoacidosis levels. In type 1 diabetics, the ketones can be produced in excessive amounts, causing the acid level of the blood to become extreme due to the body's inability to produce insulin to regulate the ketone production.

Myth #4 - Keto Causes Chronic Inflammation

The main ketone that is produced in ketosis is bHB, which has been proven to block the NLRP3 inflammasome receptor. The NLRP inflammasome reacts quickly to threats like infections, toxins, and too much glucose. By entering into ketosis, you are by definition lowering your glucose intake and cutting out many of the inflammatory foods. The ketogenic diet has been proven to lower inflammation versus increasing it.

Myth #5 - Keto Causes Muscle Loss/ You Can't Build Muscle on Keto

It is frequently claimed that keto causes a significant loss of muscle as the body recruits amino acids from muscle protein to maintain blood glucose through gluconeogenesis. It is true that the body does convert protein to make glucose to maintain blood glucose levels. The body recycles hundreds of grams of broken-down protein daily from gut cells and normal cell death. In addition to the excess protein floating around the body, you are consuming up to 150 grams of protein a day on a ketogenic diet. There is plenty of protein for the body to pull from first before ever touching muscle cells to meet its glucose needs. In reality, bHB actually decreases leucine oxidation and promotes protein synthesis.[14]

12 https://academic.oup.com/jcem/article/85/5/1963/2660569
13 https://pubmed.ncbi.nlm.nih.gov/12174324/
14 https://www.ncbi.nlm.nih.gov/pmc/articles/PMC1373635/#B6

EXERCISE IS ANOTHER ARENA IN WHICH POPULAR MYTH EXCEEDS SCIENTIFIC KNOWLEDGE. WE HAVE MANY IDEAS ABOUT HOW TO EXERCISE THAT ARE TOTALLY INGRAINED IN US THAT HAVE NO BASIS IN SCIENTIFIC FACT.

CHAPTER 2: THE KETOGENIC DIET

THE MAGIC OF KETO

If you have chosen* The Keto Coach *from the many keto diet books available to you, you probably want the basic how-to keto guide without wading through tables and tables of data or a hundred pages of scientific theory. This is the chapter where you get the magic.

In this chapter, I will explain, starting day one, how you begin a ketogenic diet. This includes:

* How do you know if you are in ketosis?
* What foods are part of a keto diet?
* Can you eat out and eat keto?
* How will you feel the first few weeks on the keto diet?
* What kind of weight loss can you expect?
* Can you cheat on your keto diet?

Measuring Your Ketones to See if You Are in Ketosis

Part of eating a keto diet is being able to effectively measure whether or not you are in ketosis (this becomes more complicated down the line for reasons I will identify later).

There are three ways to measure ketones.

PEE STRIPS

You can measure ketones in the urine (ketones are an acid, the chemical result of fat being turned into energy in your liver). This is one of the cheapest methods, but it is also very inaccurate. As you become more fat-adapted, the body will excrete less ketones in urine as it has learned how to burn those ketones as fuel. So, you might still be in ketosis but are not registering on the strips. Any brand works fine if this is your preferred method.

BREATH METERS

Several devices have been tested over the last few years. At the time of writing, the first real commercial test just hit the market. I used this device for a little over a year, but then went back to blood testing.

The breath meter was all over the place with measurements and didn't match my blood readings. In addition, it needed to be calibrated every two weeks and have the sensor replaced once a month. You lose a day of tracking your stats every time you have to power down and recalibrate the device.

BLOOD METERS

Measuring ketones in the blood is by far the most accurate method. These devices have been out for a few years now and are the preferred method for serious keto followers. I understand that some people might have an aversion to a blood meter, but this is essentially painless. My kids will even use them after meals to test their blood sugar levels for fun.

Blood ketones are best measured on a fasted stomach in the morning (before breakfast, that is). Here are a few pointers on how to interpret the result *[FIG 2.1]*.

* Below 0.5 mmol/L is not considered "ketosis," although a value of, say, 0.2 demonstrates that you're getting close. At this level, you're far away from maximum fat burning.
* Between 0.5–1.5 mmol/L is light nutritional ketosis. You'll be getting a good effect on your weight in terms of weight loss, but it's not optimal. There's more fine-tuning you can be doing with your diet.
* Around 1.5–3 mmol/L is what's called **optimal ketosis** and is recommended for maximum

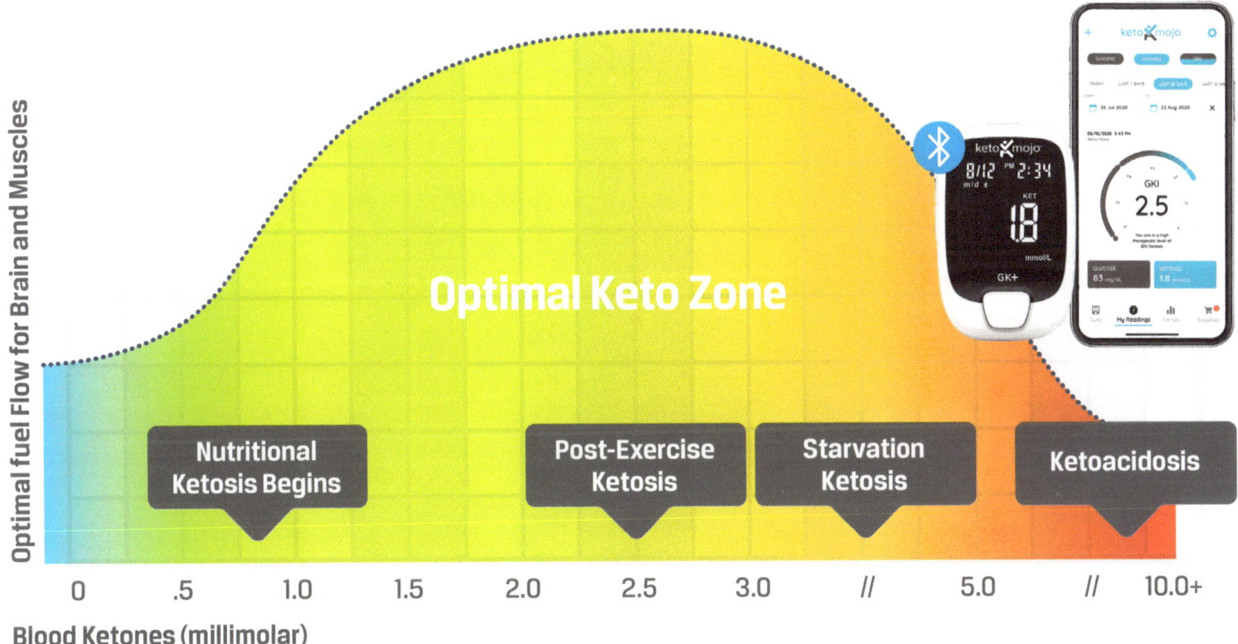

Graph data reference from: *The Art and Science of Low Carb Performance* by Phinney and Volek

FIG 2.1 ***Keto Mojo***

weight loss. This is the sweet spot: right where I want the people I am coaching. Here you get weight loss in addition to getting all the great health benefits like reducing inflammation.

* Numbers of over 3 mmol/L aren't necessary. That is, they will achieve neither better nor worse results than being at the 1.5-3 level. Higher numbers can also sometimes mean that you're not getting enough food. For type 1 diabetics, this can be caused by a severe lack of insulin (see below).
* 3-6 mmol/L is described as the therapeutic range, meant as a medical intervention and usually supervised by doctors. This is the deep stages of ketosis and is generally achieved by fasting.
* Over 8-10 mmol/l: It's normally impossible to get to this level just by eating a keto diet, and it may mean that something is wrong. The most common cause by far for this range is type 1 diabetes, with inability to produce adequate insulin. Symptoms include feeling very sick with nausea, vomiting, abdominal pain, and confusion. The possible end result, ketoacidosis, may be fatal and requires immediate medical care. These symptoms should not be confused with the "keto flu." If you have been diagnosed with type 1 diabetes, have a history of blood sugar-related ailments, or suspect that type 1 diabetes may be the cause, it is advised that you speak with your health care provider immediately, especially before starting a keto diet.
* Note that ketoacidosis is when ketones in type 1 diabetics reach levels of 20 mmol/L accompanied by a very high glucose level. For non-type 1 diabetics, your glucose level will drop as your ketone levels go up. You will likely never see levels over 6 mmol/L, as the body regulates ketone level just as it does blood sugar level.[15 16]

If you have any pre-existing medical conditions in general, you should always have your primary health care provider approve of any dietary changes (such as carbohydrate restriction).

Be aware that most blood meters were originally made for diabetics, so you will see all kinds of warnings on them that aren't relevant for people who aren't diabetic because non diabetics are able to regulate their insulin. Diabetics will have both high ketones and high insulin, which is a dangerous situation.

15 https://www.dietdoctor.com/low-carb/ketosis
16 *The Art and Science of Low Carb Performance*; p 91

GKI

In addition to measuring ketones, a new measurement has become popular in recent years: glucose ketones index, or GKI. GKI measures both your glucose and also your ketones (hence the name). This is a much more accurate and holistic way to understand what your body is doing.

I like to think of your body like a hybrid car. It can run on either the electric motor or the combustion engine. But which are you running on? Most cars will give you data on what that breakdown is. GKI is similar. Are you burning glucose or fat? In what proportion? GKI will tell you your fuel sources.

The GKI is as follows:

GKI (glucose ketone index)

* Measure both glucose and ketones
* GKI = Glucose /18 / ketones [17]
* Range
  - **<1:** Therapeutic range that can shrink tumors
  - **1-5:** Ideal fat burning range
  - **>5:** Most likely not burning fat and using glucose for fuel

Example A:
Glucose measurement = 91 mg/dL
Ketone measurement = 0.4 mmol/L
GKI = (91/18) / 0.4 = 12.6 -> burning mostly glucose for fuel

Example B:
Glucose measurement = 70 mg/dL
Ketone measurement = 1.0 mmol/L
GKI = (70/18) / 1.0 = 3.8 -> burning mostly fat for fuel

Using GKI really helped me understand my blood measurements.

One more note: you will see higher levels of glucose in the body in the morning. This is called the "dawn effect."

As the body prepares for morning, it releases glucose and cortisol into the body. It is possible to see a rise in your glucose level in the morning even if you didn't eat the day before. The body is preparing for the day by getting fuel in the blood stream.

17 The reason for the division of 18 on glucose is to move from mg/dL to mmol/L

DIET SPECIFICS

The high-level breakdown of the keto diet is as follows:

Macros

* 70% fat
* 25% protein (.5 to 1gram per 1 pounds of body weight)
* 5% carbs (20 gram or less to start)

The ketogenic diet is a low-carb, high-fat (LCHF) diet. As we have read so far, carbohydrates are fattening us up and leading us to develop metabolic syndrome. By restricting carbohydrates in the diet to less than 20 grams per day and also not overeating protein, we allow the body to transition metabolic states from glucose to ketosis. This unlocks the body's ability to burn fat and heal itself.

Once on an LCHF diet, you will naturally want to eat less (really!). Your hunger pains will disappear once the body has learned to use its body fat again, making it easier to accelerate your weight loss progress.

One key part of the ketogenic diet is **fat**. If you were to combine a low carb and low-fat diet, you would starve. The trick on the keto diet is to: 1) eat only when hungry, and 2) to eat more fat to help you feel satisfied.

For example, just try to eat eight slices of full fat cheddar cheese. I bet you can't. The body will signal you that you are full after few pieces, unlike the carbs that never fill you up. It is important at the beginning of your diet that you

One key part of the ketogenic diet is fat. If you were to combine a low carb and low-fat diet, you would starve.

don't feel hungry to help you stick with the plan. That's the magic (or really, the science) of keto: you will lose weight without cutting calories.

A ketogenic diet is primarily made up of "real food," not specially created, store-bought, low-carb products. If you were in the grocery store, this would be only the outside aisles and avoiding all the processed foods in the middle aisles. When you think real food, this means fish, meat, eggs, butter, above-ground vegetables, olive oil, bacon, nuts ... Not grains, pasta, bread, rice, anything in a box, sugar, heavy beers, or sodas.

The good news is that all your fantasies of binging on real butter, heavy whipping cream, and bacon are about to come true. Who needs Twinkies when you can have steak every day?

For many people, eating this way runs counter to everything they have ever been taught (as we covered in the introduction). It can take some time to get over the mental hurdle of putting full fat or highly salted foods in your mouth. But you will be surprised by how good you feel once your body has adjusted.

We aren't reinventing the wheel here. There are cultures that already eat this way. In fact, the best example of this is called the "French Paradox." French food culture is heavy in cream, fatty cheese, red meat, red wine, and all other kinds of treats, and yet the French are notoriously slender and have low rates of heart disease and other metabolic diseases. It's almost as if we are meant to eat this way *[FIG 2.2]*.

www.dietdoctor.com/low-carb/keto

A fundamental tenet of keto is to eat less than 20 grams of carbs per day to start to get into fat-burning mode. Counting the grams in your carbs will become second-nature, but for now, the following pages are a guide to get you started *[FIG 2.3, 2.4]*.

FOODS TO EAT:

Meat

Fish

Eggs and bacon

Vegetables
(avocadoes are amazing)

Natural fats
(use real butter and cream, conconut oil, olive oil, real whole fat cheese, high-fat yogurt–like greek yogurt)

Nuts
(cashews, macadamia nuts)

Berries
(in small portions–up to 5 a day)

FOODS TO AVOID:

Potatoes, carrots

Low-fat products
(they replace the fat with sugar)

Sugar, rice, and starches

Pasta

Fruit juice and soda

Beer
(you can drink low-carb beer like Ultra or Miller Lite)

Fruit
(berries are the exception)

"Middle of the Store"
(most everything is in a box or a can)

Anything "low-fat"
(foods have fat in them naturally; to get rid of the fat they add carbohydrates in its place. Just look at the label between the full fat version and low fat and notice the difference in carbs)

FIG 2.2 ***Foods to Eat***

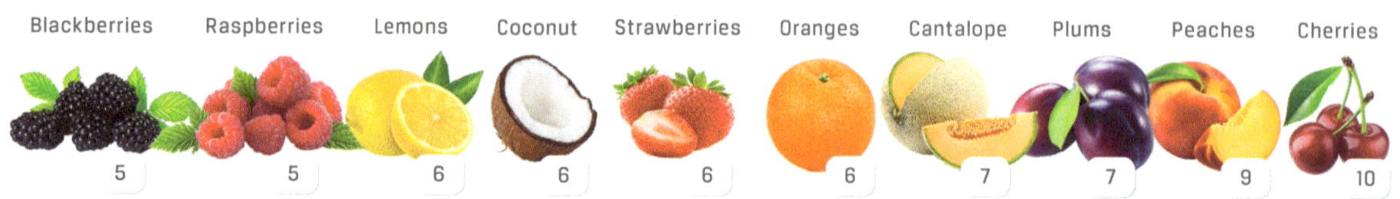

Blackberries
5
Raspberries
5
Lemons
6
Coconut
6
Strawberries
6
Oranges
6
Cantalope
7
Plums
7
Peaches
9
Cherries
10

FRUITS

Celery
1
Spinach
1
Lettuce
2
Avocado
2
Asparagus
2
Olives
3
Zuccini
3
Cucumber
3

VEGETABLES

Beet Root
7
Carrots
7
Celeriac
7
Onions
7

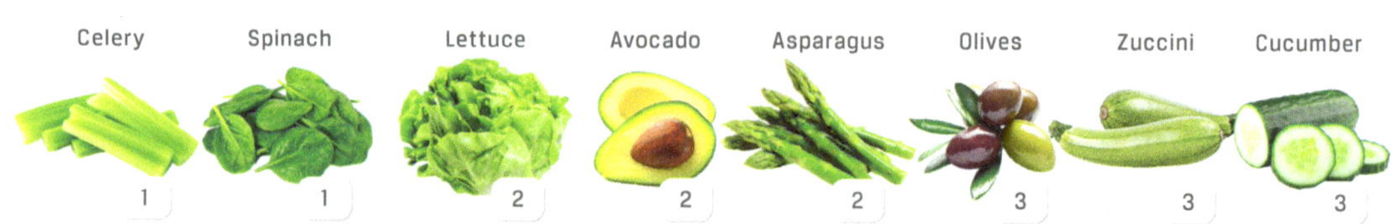

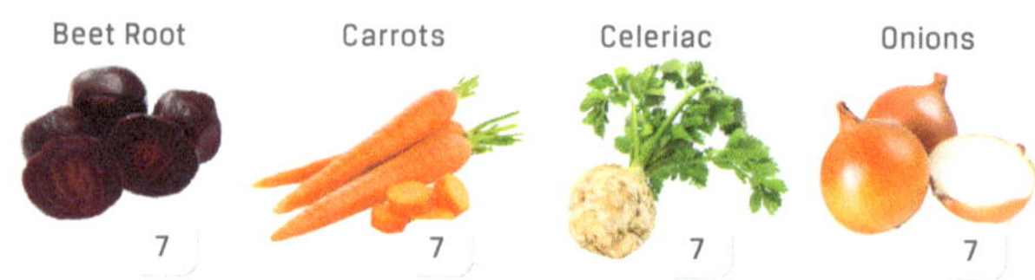

ROOTS

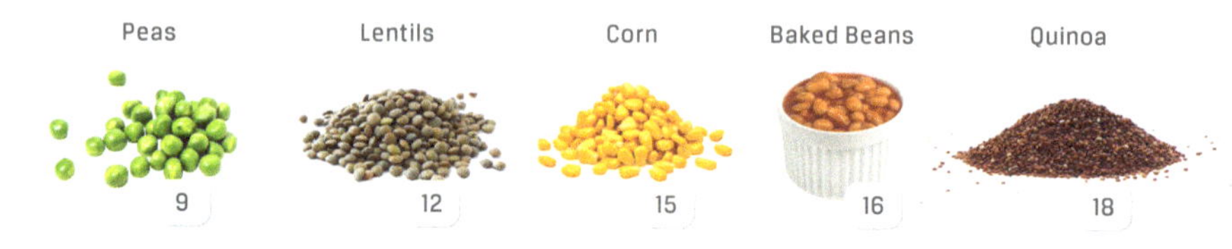

LENTILS / GRAINS / BREADS

Brazil Nuts
4
Macadamia
5
Peanuts
7
Hazel Nuts
7
Pecans
7

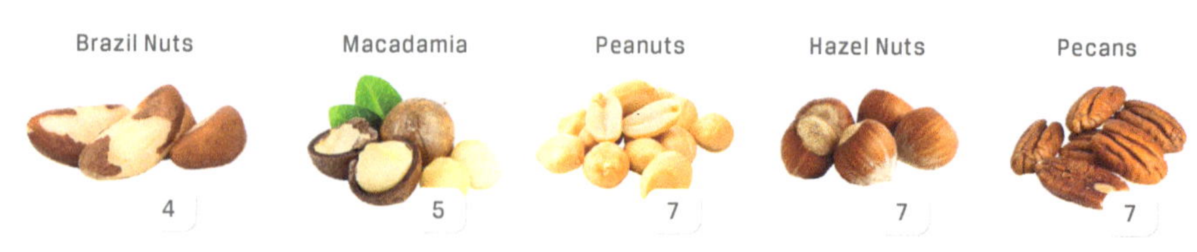

NUTS

‹ **LESS CARBS**

FIG 2.3 ***Diet Doctor Food Spectrum*** ***All amounts estimated*

Watermelon 10
Clementines 10
Blueberries 12
Pears 12
Pineapple 12
Kiwi 12
Apples 12
Mangos 13
Grapes 16
Bananas 20

Cabbage 3
Tomatoes 3
Eggplant 3
Peppers 3,4,5
Kale 4
Broccoli 4
Cauliflower 4
Brussel Sprouts 5

Rutabaga 7
Parsnips 13
Potatoes 15
Sweet Potatoes 17

Rice 28
Pasta 29
Bread 46
Donut 49
Cookies 58

Walnuts 7
Pine Nuts 9
Almonds 10
Pistachios 18
Cashews 27

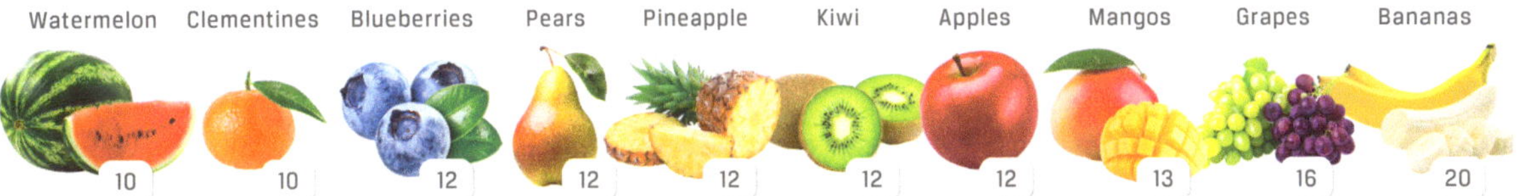

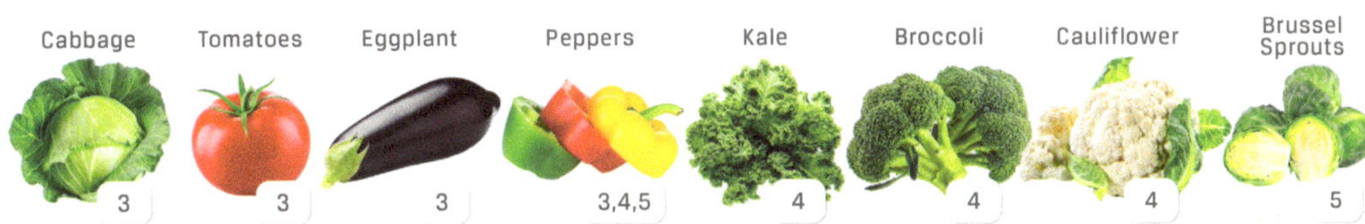

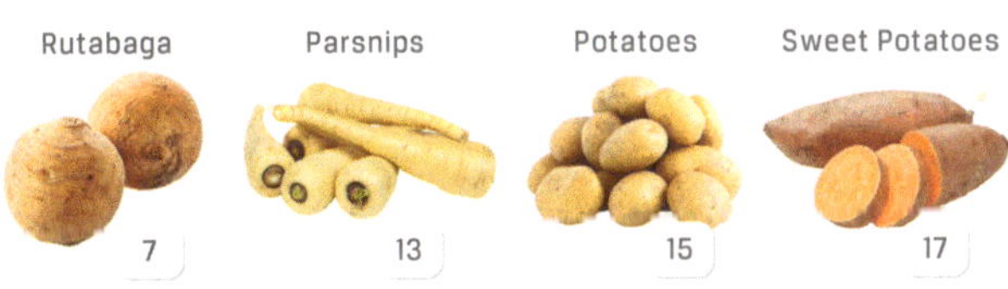

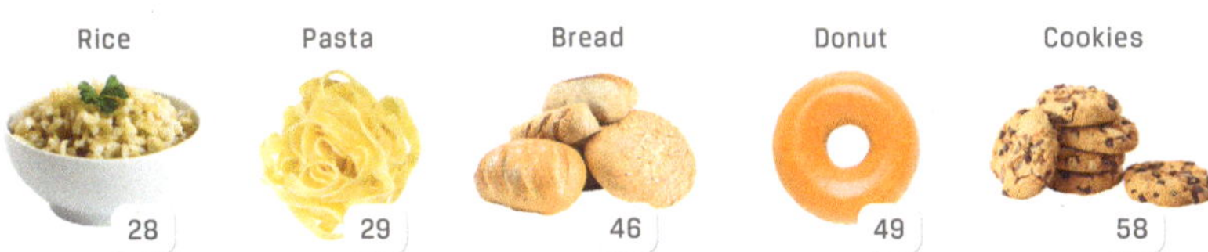

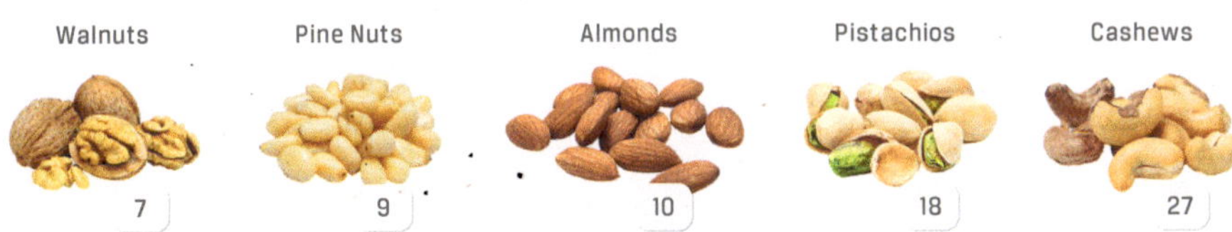

MORE CARBS ›

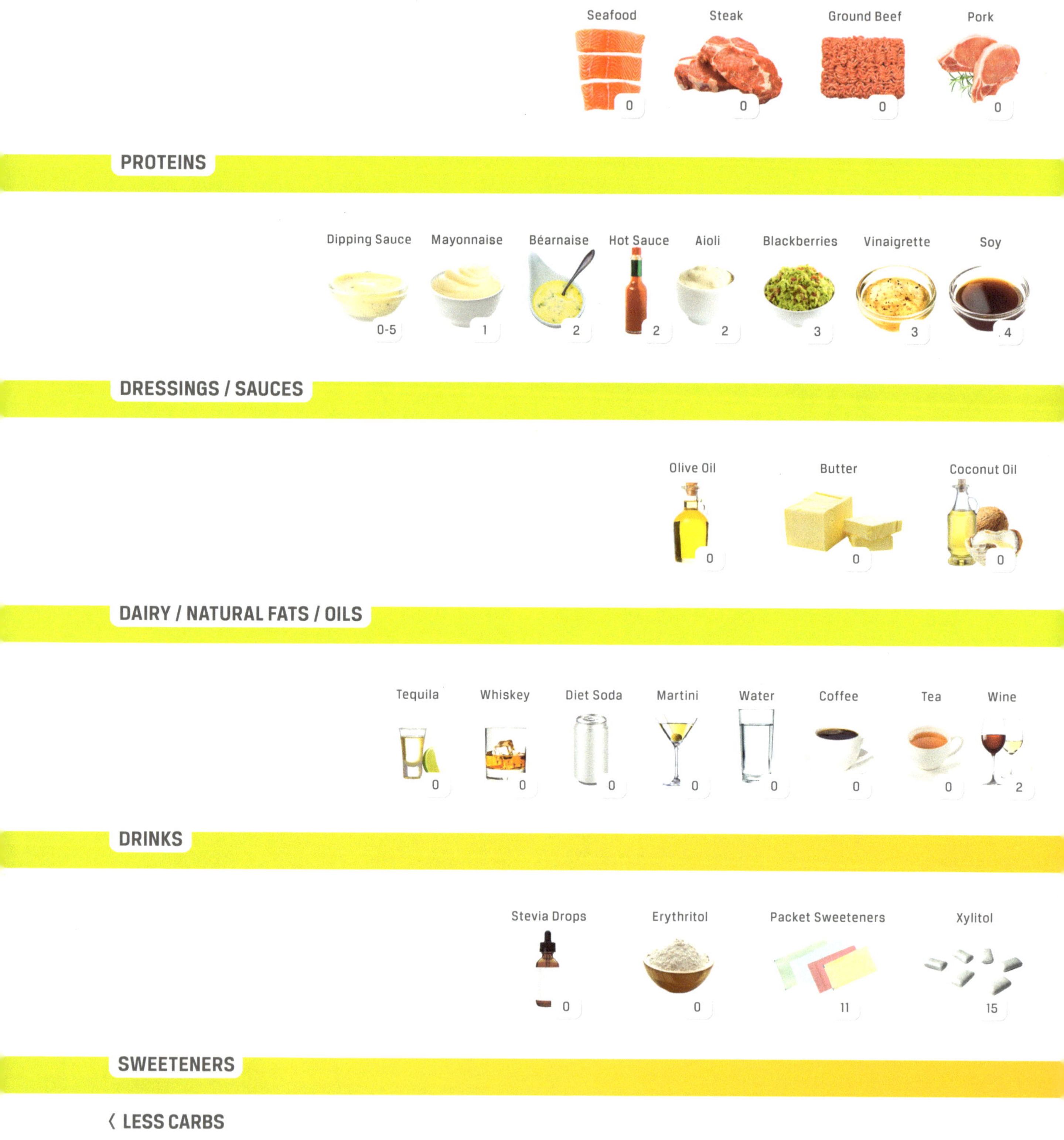

Seafood
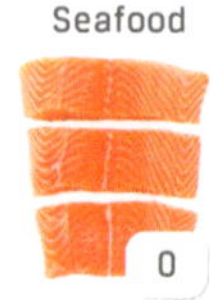
0

Steak
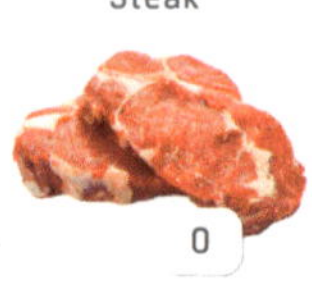
0

Ground Beef
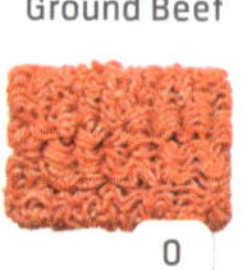
0

Pork
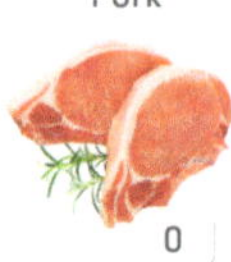
0

PROTEINS

Dipping Sauce
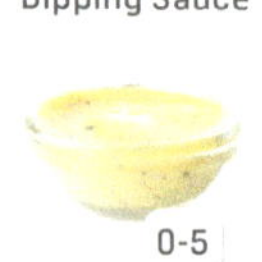
0-5

Mayonnaise
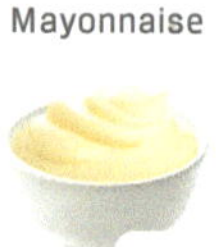
1

Béarnaise
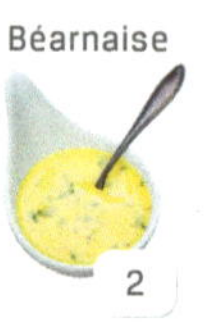
2

Hot Sauce
2

Aioli
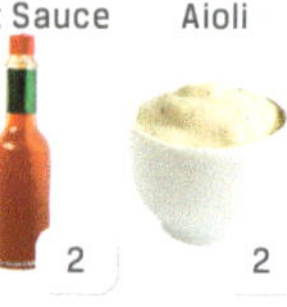
2

Blackberries
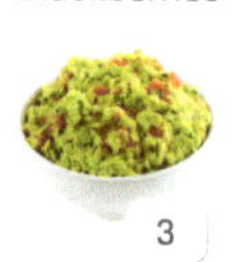
3

Vinaigrette
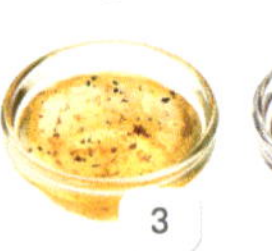
3

Soy
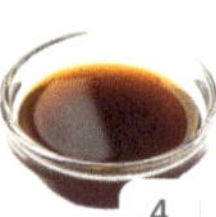
4

DRESSINGS / SAUCES

Olive Oil
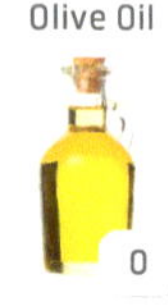
0

Butter
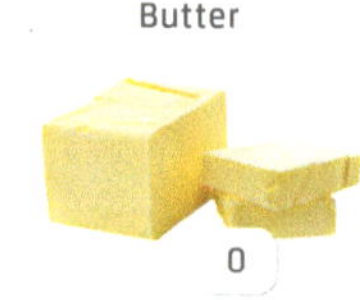
0

Coconut Oil
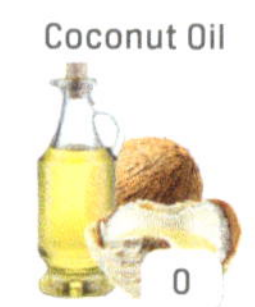
0

DAIRY / NATURAL FATS / OILS

Tequila
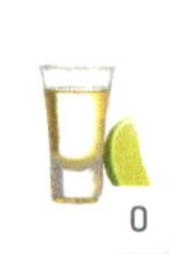
0

Whiskey
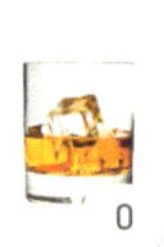
0

Diet Soda
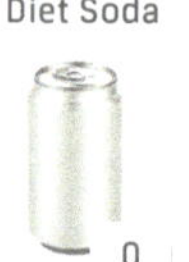
0

Martini
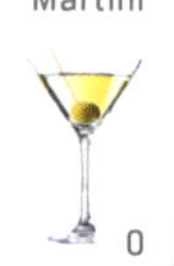
0

Water
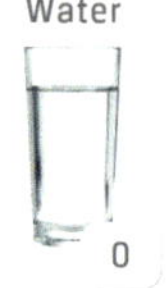
0

Coffee
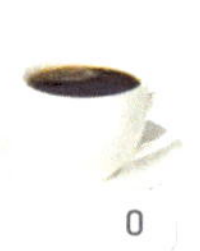
0

Tea
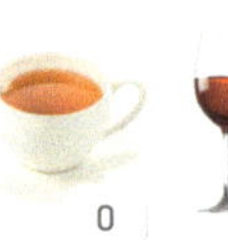
0

Wine
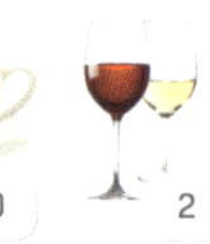
2

DRINKS

Stevia Drops
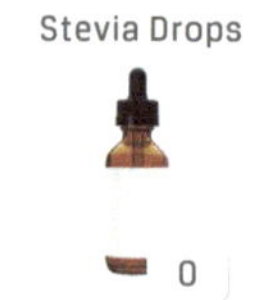
0

Erythritol
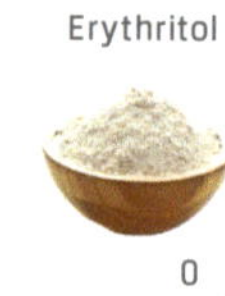
0

Packet Sweeteners
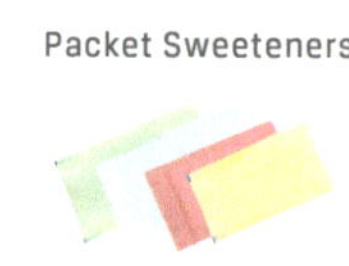
11

Xylitol
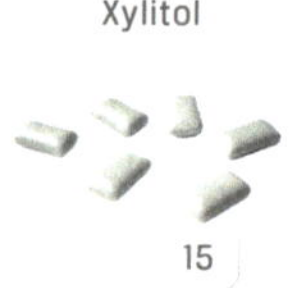
15

SWEETENERS

‹ LESS CARBS

FIG 2.4 ***Diet Doctor Food Spectrum*** **All amounts estimated*

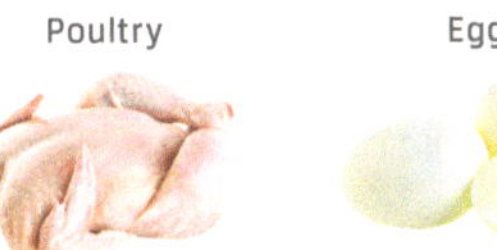

Poultry	Eggs	Cold Cuts
0	1	2

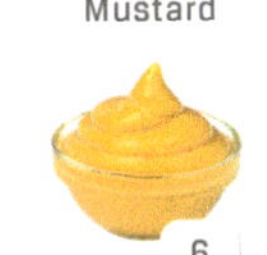
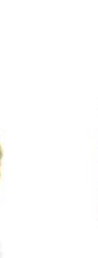
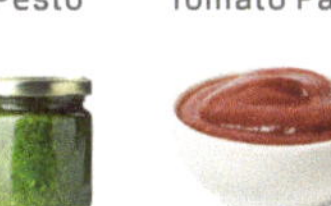
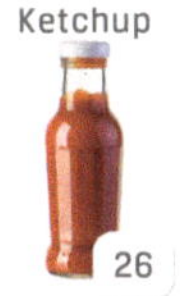
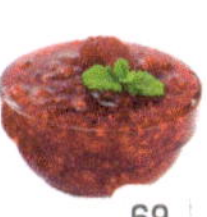

Salsa	Mustard	Pesto	Tomato Paste	Ketchup	Barbeque	Preserves
6	6	8	15	26	40	69

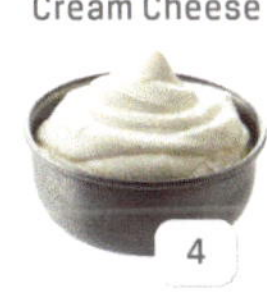
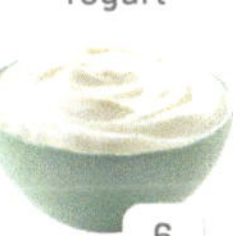

Cheese	Cream	Cream Cheese	Yogurt
2	3	4	6

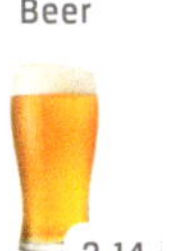
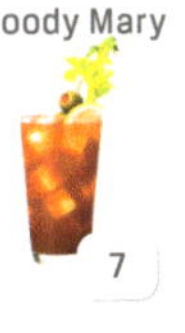
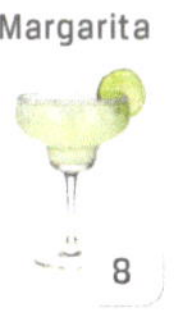
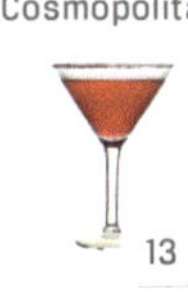
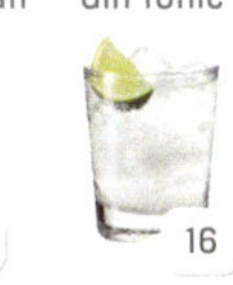
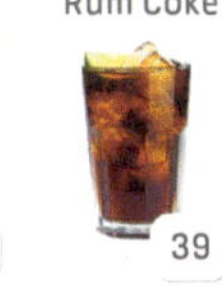
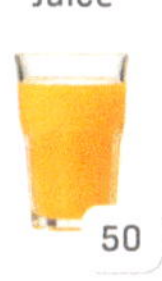
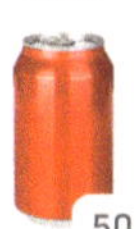

Beer	Bloody Mary	Margarita	Cosmopolitan	Gin Tonic	Rum Coke	Juice	Soda
2-14	7	8	13	16	39	50	50

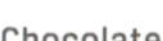
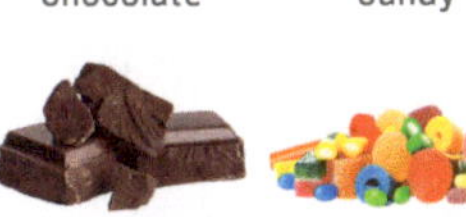
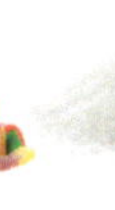
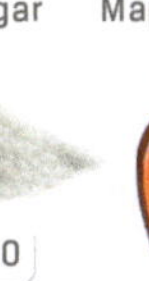
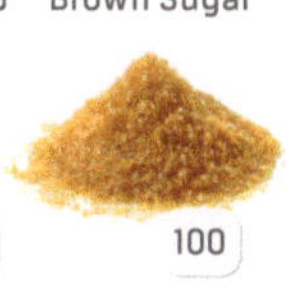
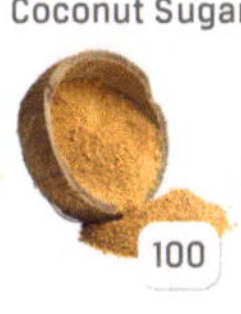
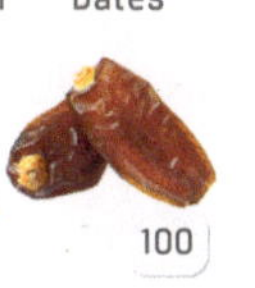
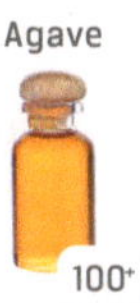
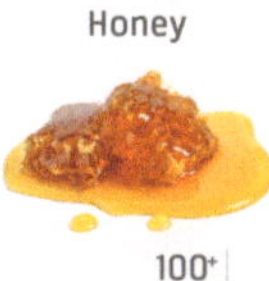

Chocolate	Candy	White Sugar	Maple Syrup	Brown Sugar	Coconut Sugar	Dates	Agave	Honey
60	70	100	100	100	100	100	100+	100+

MORE CARBS ›

Gluconeogenesis: Too Much Protein in One Meal Is Bad

Remember: you can overdo it on the protein.

People often assume that keto is an all-meat diet, but that isn't true. Keto isn't a protein-unlimited diet. It's high *fat*, not high protein. This is because of what happens when you eat excess protein.

Gluconeogenesis is the process in which protein is converted back to sugar if glucose levels get too low. The liver can then break down protein to generate glucose to bring blood sugar levels back to normal.

The recommended protein ratios are between 0.5 grams to 1 gram per pound of muscle weight.

To find your muscle weight, simply weigh yourself and subtract the fat weight.

Example: 180lbs with 20% fat. 180 x 20% = 36,
180lbs is 36lbs of fat = 144lbs of muscle

144lbs of muscle x 0.7 grams of protein
= 100.8 grams of protein a day

The rest of diet should be made up of fats.

The body is able to recycle 300g of protein a day from broken-down cells.

The body can't consume more than 35g of protein in a single hour. The excess protein can't be stored, so the body will convert the excess protein to glucose.

What I'm really trying to say is that gluconeogenesis is the process where protein gets converted into glucose. The body can only digest 30 grams of protein in a single meal. You should only have 100 grams of protein a day if you're having 3 meals a day. Add a fourth meal if you require more protein.

Remember: a ketogenic diet is high fat, moderate protein, and low carb.

Sugar Is Toxic

The current consumption level of sugar in the US is at levels toxic to the body. It has an outsized contribution to weight gain and the ripple effects that drive metabolic syndrome.

Sugar comes in many forms:

TABLE SUGAR

Table sugar is technically half glucose and half fructose.

In the early 1900s, sugar was hailed because of its low caloric count. As I have proven, we now know that calories have little to do with gaining or losing weight. Table sugar and most sugars added to manufactured products are highly refined to get them to the pure form we see today. This means that there is no fiber in them, so they are absorbed by the body very quickly and do not send a signal to the brain that you are full.

The fructose in sugar is even more dangerous. Fructose was once thought to be a better sweetener than table sugar because it did not raise blood sugar. What we didn't know then was that, unlike the glucose portion of sugar that all cells of the body can burn, fructose can only be processed in the liver.

So, if you weigh 180 pounds, 1 gram of glucose from sugar has all 180 pounds of your mass to consume it since it can be processed in any cell. 1 gram of fructose only has all 3 pounds of your liver mass to burn it. The liver can only burn a small amount of that 1 gram of fructose and then has to store the rest as fat on the liver. The liver is not designed to store fat like adipose tissue (belly fat). This is known as non-alcoholic fatty liver disease, which causes metabolic syndrome.

High-fructose corn syrup was and is a cheap way to add sugar to foods. When the low-fat craze started, fat was removed from products and replaced with high-fructose corn syrup to make the low-fat food taste better. HFCS-55 is 55% fructose and 45% glucose. Honestly, this is not really any worse than regular table sugar, but it is *all* bad at the levels we are eating them today.

FRUIT

It is important that we discuss fruit, which we widely consider to be a "healthy" snack. Truth is: it is not. Even though fruit is rich in wonderful micro-nutrients, eating too much fruit makes you fat.

Why? Modern day fruit has been bred to be much sweeter than what nature produced. Fruit also was naturally eaten only when it was in season: at the end of summer before we put on weight for the coming colder months. (Isn't it ironic that summer is the season for fattening?) Now we eat fruit year-round and daily, which we are not evolved to do.

In addition, current fruits bought in the store today have very high levels of fructose in them. Unlike glucose, fructose can *only* be digested in the liver, thus limiting how much of the energy from fruit we can actually use versus how much we store as fat. 1 gram of fructose is not equal to

1 gram of glucose, as fructose does *not* trigger leptin. Keep in mind that the natural version of fruit has half the sugar of modern fruit and much more fiber, allowing for the sugar to be absorbed slower.

The worst thing we are doing to our kids is giving them fruit juice, like orange juice. It is terrible for them—just cups of sugar. Even modern-day juicing diets with fresh fruit isn't good. Ideally, you would throw away the juice and just keep the pulp. That is where all the good stuff is.

This runs counter to plenty of diet advice, but be wary of fruit-heavy diets, particularly those that involve grinding up multiple bananas a day to throw in things like protein shakes. Bananas have 18.5 grams of carbs in one small banana. There is a reason you are not losing any weight on those diets!

HONEY AND MAPLE SYRUP

Honey and maple syrup were nature's natural sugars that were consumed until cane sugar and sugar beets were discovered.

Honey is too high in sugar for us, just like fruit. There are 15 grams per serving of honey.

Maple syrup generally has tons of sugar added to it:

53 grams of sugar added!

A good alternative is Lakanto Maple Syrup:

1 net carb - 9 carbs total, 3 from fiber and 5 from sugar alcohol - so 9-3-5 = 1 net carbs

I use this with my kids, and they think it has more sugar than regular syrup.

Keto Vegetarians and Vegans

Keto is commonly interpreted to be an all *meat* diet, but this is far from true. While keto cuts carbs and focuses more on proteins, it is also not a high protein diet. When you eat keto, you should be eating a generous portion of leafy greens every day.

It is entirely possible to eat a vegetarian keto diet. By replacing the meat with vegetarian protein options like beans or tofu (be careful of this one—you want to avoid tofu because it's made from soy. While its macros might work, soy is highly inflammatory to the body. Also, most soy is GMO, which means it will affect the thyroid and cause issues with leaky gut and autoimmune disease), you should be in good shape. Eggs are also an excellent source of protein for vegetarians and non-vegetarians alike.

If you are attempting to eat keto and vegan, this is a much more complicated challenge; however, a growing online movement offers great recipes and nutritional tips. Plenty of good plant-based fat sources, like avocados, are widely available.

Sourcing Your Food

In my time coaching, I have heard concerns from some people that eating keto can be expensive. It's true that mass produced, processed food can be cheaper than organic produce and meats. The unfortunate truth is that you are often paying a premium for food that isn't injected with hormones or covered in pesticides.

HONEY
SERVING SIZE: 1 tbsp
TOTAL CARBS: 17g
SUGARS: 15g

MAPLE SYRUP
SERVING SIZE: 4 tbsp
TOTAL CARBS: 53g
SUGARS: 53g

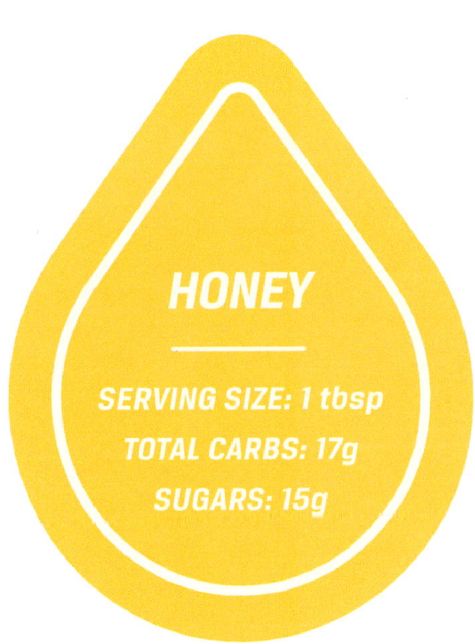

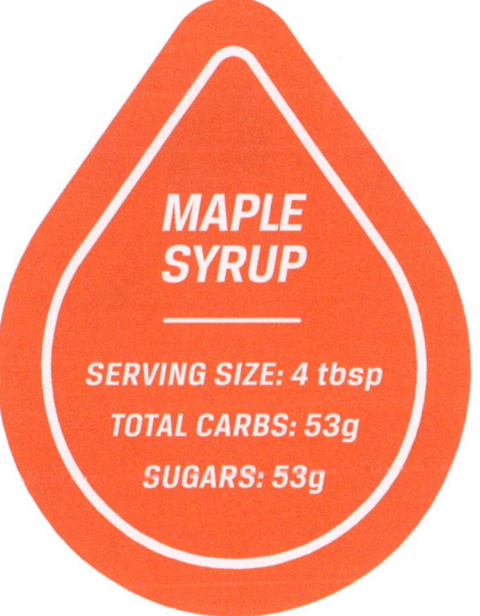

I believe that it is worth it to pay more for quality food; after all, whatever money you save on cheaper food, you're making up the difference in your health. I also have found that cost is another issue that can be mitigated by advance planning.

For example, organic produce can be fairly affordably obtained at supermarkets. Meat can be a different issue. Eating a steak a day is expensive, and if that beef is free-range and hormone-free, you're really going to be paying.

But, there are excellent services out there that can help you offset this cost. My family and I use one called Butcherbox that delivers high quality meat in bulk in a monthly delivery. Not only is this cost effective, it also cuts down the amount of time I am spending either in the grocery store or planning meals.

When you buy food in advance, make batches of meals, and freeze what you are not eating in the moment, you can effectively manage keto on a budget. There are many fancy keto snacks (ones I happen to use and love) that can be pre-packaged. Bars, desserts, and the like. These can also be bought in bulk or recreated at home for a fraction of the cost.

Plus, how do you put a number on the value of your health? What would you pay to minimize the risk of contracting fatal diseases later in life? What would you pay to quickly and healthily shed 45 pounds?

Meal Prep

How many times have you adopted a diet only to later abandon it? The key to sticking to the new lifestyle is follow the Boy Scout Motto, "Be prepared."

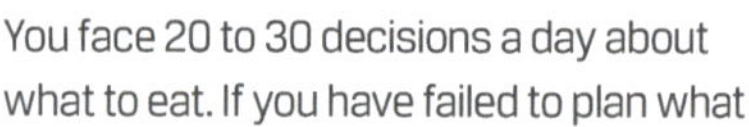

You face 20 to 30 decisions a day about what to eat. If you have failed to plan what to eat, you will eat what is available. Fast food and junk food are everywhere and easy to find. Ketogenic food is harder to come by at first glance.

I recommend preparing your meals twice a week to keep yourself from being unprepared. Also, when cooking dinner, make two portions: one for dinner and one for lunch the following day.

SUNDAY MEAL PREP

The key to meal prep is to knock it all out in 2 hours and get lots of meals for the week. First order yourself the following:

Glass meal prep food storage containers (6-pack 28 oz.); portion control lunch containers with BPA-free airtight snap locking lids; prep, freeze, reheat and bake oven-safe containers for home and work

To speed up cooking:

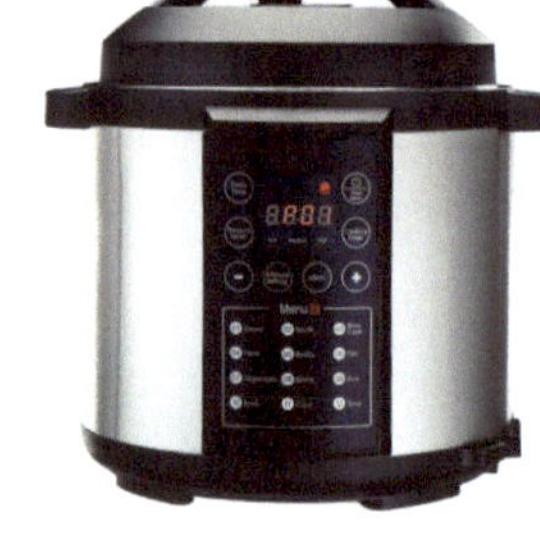

INSTAPOT

Instant Pot DUO Plus-8 Qt. 9-in-1 Multi-Use Programmable Pressure Cooker, Slow Cooker, Rice Cooker, Yogurt Maker, Egg Cooker, Sauté, Steamer, Warmer, and Sterilizer

More recipes will follow in the back. This is just the plan to get you started on your first week of keto.

Prepare a casserole in the oven for breakfast and then divide up into individual servings for the week:

Ensuring Successs

* *Eat only when hungry—Eat more fat to avoid starvation: olive oil, fatty fish, avocado, nuts*
* *Drink lots of caffeine throughout the day to increase metabolism and burn 2x fat*
* *Eat protein after workout to speed up fat burning*
* *Eat plain tuna in oil to curb hunger: the oil gets you to the right macros*
* *Exercise 30 minutes a day to keep metabolism up*
* *Lift weights to keep from losing muscle*
* *Sleep 8 hours: lack of sleep causes stress (cortisol)*

MENU PREP SAMPLE:

Meal #1: Breakfast Casserole

Ingredients:

* 1 lb. ground beef (80/20)
* 12 large eggs
* 4 oz. cheddar cheese
* ¼ cup heavy cream
* 5 cups fresh spinach
* 1 tsp pink salt
* ½ tsp black pepper

Instructions:

* Heat oven to 350
* Cook ground beef on stove then add spinach to pan for a few minutes
* Mix eggs with heavy cream and salt and pepper
* Put ground beef with spinach in a casserole pan and pour egg mixture over
* Bake 30-40 minutes

Meal # 2: Keto Crack Chicken Instant Pot

Ingredients:

* 2 lbs. chicken
* 1 Tbsp of dry chives
* ½ cup of water
* 2 Tbsp apple cider vinegar
* 4 bacon strips
* 2 blocks of cream cheese
* 1 Tbsp of onion powder
* 1 Tbsp of garlic powder
* ¼ tsp of salt and pepper

Instructions:

* Place your Instant Pot on sauté and add cut-up bacon. Cook 3-5 minutes until brown
* Add 2 pounds of chicken, salt & pepper, cream cheese, onion powder, and garlic powder, dry chives, apple cider vinegar
* Seal Instant pot and cook on high pressure for 20 minutes
* Remove lid after venting steam and set Instant pot to keep warm
* Shred the chicken with a fork and put back in pot, stir well, and let sit for 2 minutes
* Divide up into 6 individual meals

MENU PREP SAMPLE:

Meal #3: Keto Pesto Chicken & Cauliflower Rice

Ingredients:

* 2 pounds chicken thighs
* 2 Tbsp avocado oil
* 3 oz. green pesto
* 1 ½ cup of heavy whipping cream
* 3 oz. pitted olives
* 6 oz. feta cheese
* 1 Tbsp of Onion powder
* 1 Tbsp of Garlic powder
* ¼ tsp of Salt and pepper
* 1 bag of cauliflower rice

Instructions:

* Place your Instant Pot on sauté and add chicken and avocado oil. Cook 3-5 minutes until brown
* Add green pesto, salt & pepper, heavy whipping cream, onion powder, and garlic powder, olives, and feta
* Add one bag of cauliflower rice
* Seal Instant pot and cook on high pressure for 25 minutes
* Remove lid after venting steam and set Instant pot to keep warm
* Divide up into 6 individual meals

Meal # 4: Instant Pot Beef Brisket

Ingredients:

* 3 lbs. beef brisket
* Rub
    - 1 Tbsp ground cumin
    - 1 Tbsp paprika
    - 1 Tbsp garlic powder
    - 2 Tbsp pink Himalayan salt
    - 1 Tbsp ground black pepper
* Braise
    - 2 Tbsp avocado oil
    - 1 diced onion
    - ¼ cup tomato paste
    - ¼ cup balsamic vinegar
    - ¼ cup whole grain mustard seed
    - 2 cups water

Instructions:

* Mix rub together and heavily coat each side of the brisket
* Place your Instant Pot on sauté and add Brisket and avocado oil. Cook 3-5 minutes until brown
* Add onion, tomato paste, balsamic vinegar, mustard seed, water
* Seal Instant pot and cook on high pressure for 70 minutes
* Remove lid after venting steam and set Instant pot to keep warm
* Divide up into 6 individual meals
* Serve over cauliflower rice

Freeze some of the meals for later in the week.

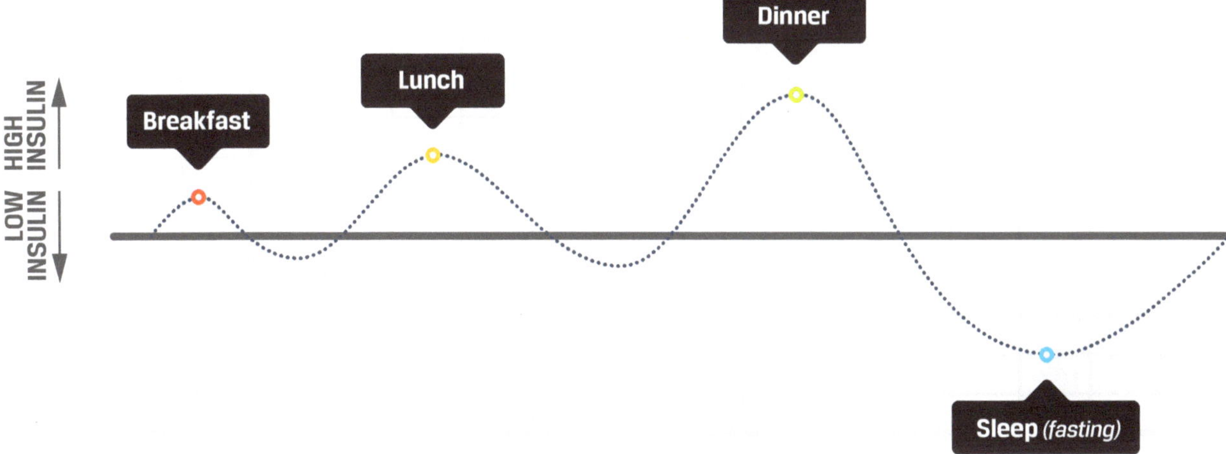

Insulin release with an eating pattern of three meals, no snacks.

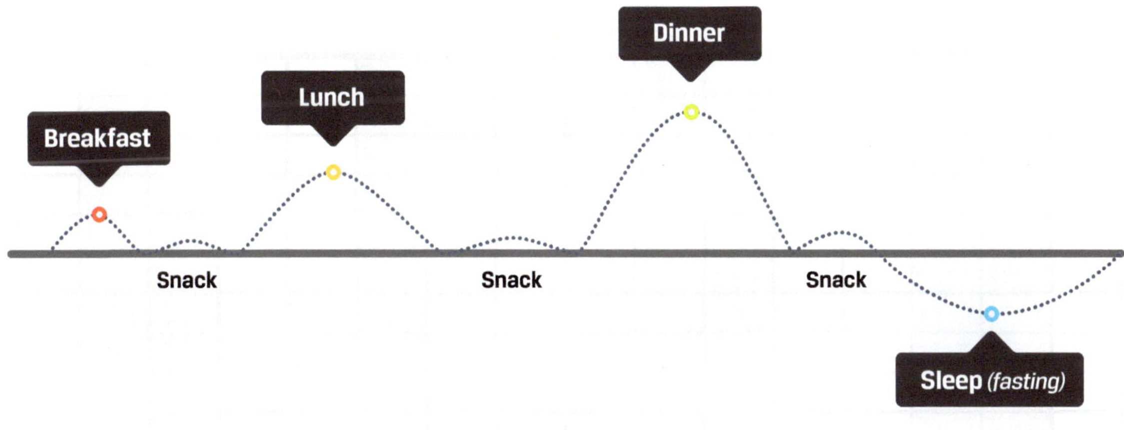

Insulin release with an eating pattern of multiple meals and snacks.

FIG 2.5 ***Insulin Release***

Eating Schedule

So, *when* do you eat on keto? Three big meals a day? One big meal in the morning? Constant snacks to keep your metabolism right?

Actually, none of this is right. When you are just beginning to eat keto, you should eat 3 meals a day on a tightly planned schedule. Reducing the number of choices you are making on keto is important. Eventually you will learn what it feels like when your body is *actually* hungry and you will eat then.

Additionally, you want to avoid snacking. Snacking keeps your insulin high all day, preventing weight loss [18] *[FIG 2.5]*.

Remember that the primary reason for the weight gain and the struggle to lose weight is caused by being insulin-resistant. We need insulin to come down between meals and overnight so that the cells become sensitive to insulin again and require the body to produce less insulin throughout the day. Once insulin goes down, the body will switch to burning fat.

18 Source Good Calories, Bad Calories by Gary Taubes

Glycaemic Load

How Much Sugar Equivalent Are You Consuming

The following chart blew my mind the first time I saw it. I never felt like I ate much sugar, but I certainly ate the foods on the chart. Eating a serving of french fries is the same as eating 7.5 teaspoons of sugar. It all gets converted into sugar in the body, no different than eating sweets *[FIG 2.6]*.

Eating at Fast Food Places

People tend to assume that eating keto means you can never eat at a restaurant again. Not true. Eating out isn't difficult on a keto diet as long as you remember your guidelines. Stick to proteins and the approved vegetables. Stay away from heavy sauces and anything bready.

Best part of a keto diet: you can even eat at fast food restaurants! Below is a guide to specific fast food restaurants and how to navigate their menus *[FIG 2.7]*.

A Night Out on Keto

If you want to have a fancy date night or celebration and are worried that you can't keep to the keto diet, here's my suggestion: start with a side salad (no croutons), and then a 6-8 ounce steak with a side of steamed broccoli or asparagus. Easy.

Keto Flu and Other Side Effects

Many people who begin a ketogenic diet experience what is known as the "keto flu." Headaches, leg cramps, constipation—anything that feels like the common flu—are symptoms. So, what's going on?

This reaction is caused by a lack of salt. That's right: salt.

As you stop eating carbs and enter ketosis, your body will no longer need all the excess water it has been storing. Your body will get rid of a massive amount of water during the first few days. Your salt is stored in this water. The body needs sodium to function; this is part of the electrolytes.[19]

Make sure that you are salting your food heavily (pink Himalayan salt preferred) and increasing your water intake.

And, as always, make sure you are getting enough fat. A low carb plus low fat diet leads to starvation and feeling tired.

Here is how to respond to the specific symptoms you are experiencing:

19 https://www.health.harvard.edu/heart-health/take-it-with-a-grain-of-salt

Food Item	Glycaemic index	Serving Size (g)	How does each serving of food affect blood glucose compared with one 4g teaspoon of table sugar?
Rice	69	150	10.1
Potato	86	150	8.2
French Fries	64	150	7.5
Spaghetti	39	180	6.6
Peas	51	80	1.3
Sweet Corn	60	80	7.3
Banana	62	120	5.7
Apple	39	120	2.3
Wholemeal	74	30	3
Broccoli	54	80	.2
Eggs	0	60	0

Source: Atkinson FS, Foster-Powell k, Brand-Miller JC. International tables of glycemic index and glycemic load values: 2008. Diabetes Care. 2008; 31(12):2281-2283. http://dx.doi.org/10.2337/dc08-1239. Table A1 where the index is greater than zero or for broccoli, which is appoximated based on available carbohydrate composition.

Fig 2.6 **Glycaemic Load**

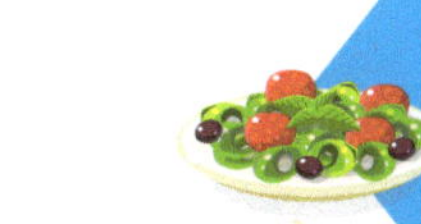

Coffee Shop
Black coffee with heavy cream
Double espresso with no sugar
Nitro cold brew with no water
You can sweeten with monk fruit or stevia

Italian Food
Fish, sausage, or steak with vegetables
"Zoodles" zucchini noodles with alfredo sauce
Chicken or salmon piccata, herb salmon
Salad; Italian dressing, ranch or blue cheese
– no croutons or carrots

Burger Joint
Burger King, McDonalds, In-N-Out Burger, 5 guys, etc.
Bacon cheeseburger with no bun or ketchup,
Add mustard, mayo, avocado or guacamole;
Served in lettuce wrap or over shredded lettuce

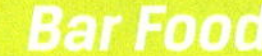

Asian Restaurants
Sauces are are high in sugar, avoid the rice
Egg drop soup is okay
Chicken lettuce wraps

Sandwich Shop
Subway, Jimmy Johns, Jersey Mike's, etc.
Order a sandwich as a salad or in a bowl
Add mayo or ranch to increase the fat content

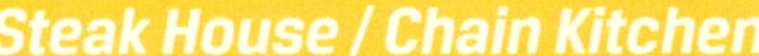

Bar Food
Cheese burger with no bun in a lettuce wrap
Non-breaded wings in buffalo sauce with
blue cheese; Cobb salad with ranch dressing
–no croutons or carrots

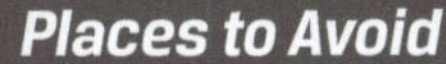

Mexican Food
Order fajitas and avoid the beans and tortillas
Taco salad with no beans, just don't eat the shell
Get tequila on the rocks–no sugar

Steak House / Chain Kitchen
6-12oz ribeye with asparagus or steamed
broccoli; Side salad with ranch or
blue cheese dressing–no croutons or carrots

Places to Avoid
Pizza Hut, KFC–nothing to eat there

FIG 2.7 ***Eating Out on Keto***

Headaches and Feeling Sluggish

If you have a headache and are feeling sluggish now (the two will generally go together), add a teaspoon of salt to a large glass of water—and enjoy! I know it sounds odd, but you should feel better in 30 minutes. Symptoms like these are typical for most during the first four days of eating keto and will pass as the body becomes fat-adapted.

Leg Cramps

If the salt and water combo don't fix leg cramps, add a daily magnesium supplement to your routine. (Slow-Mag is one I personally recommend.)

Constipation

Salt and water will cure the common cause of constipation on the low carb diet: dehydration. If you are drinking plenty of water and salt and still having trouble, make sure you have enough fiber from vegetables in your diet. The final solution would be to take Milk of Magnesia to cure the constipation. (Just be careful here to be close to a bathroom when you take it, as it may trigger diarrhea very quickly.)

Bad Breath

As we discussed in the Measuring Ketones section, the ketone body acetone can be measured on the breath. The smell can be fruity or like that of a solvent. This is a temporary phase for most people in the first few weeks while the body learns how to use the ketones being produced from fat-burning. Make sure you are drinking enough water so as to not have a dry mouth and so that your body has enough fluids to continue to flush itself.

Heart Palpitations

During the first two weeks, you may have an elevated heart rate or even heart palpitations. This is typically caused by the heart having to work harder due to dehydration and the lack of salt to increase the fluid in the blood steam.

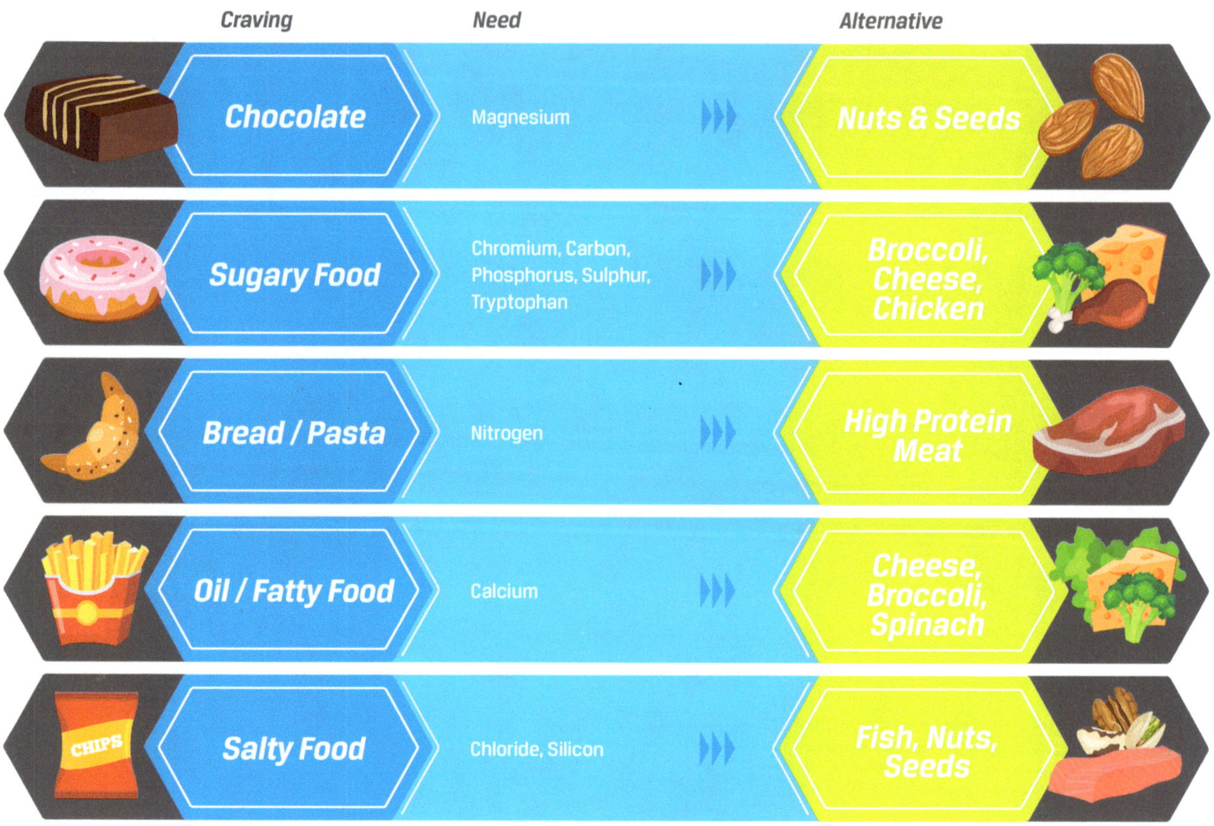

Craving	Need	Alternative
Chocolate	Magnesium	Nuts & Seeds
Sugary Food	Chromium, Carbon, Phosphorus, Sulphur, Tryptophan	Broccoli, Cheese, Chicken
Bread / Pasta	Nitrogen	High Protein Meat
Oil / Fatty Food	Calcium	Cheese, Broccoli, Spinach
Salty Food	Chloride, Silicon	Fish, Nuts, Seeds

FIG 2.8 ***What Are You Craving?***

Coldness

Coldness is caused by the lack of blood sugar in the blood stream. This is a temporary state that usually only lasts a day or two. When your ketones get above 1.5, you will feel full of energy and warm again.

Now that you are eating keto, you have changed your diet input a lot. This means you may be deficient in certain vitamins or nutrients and as a result crave certain foods. Here is a good chart to interrupt your cravings *[FIG 2.8]*.

Tracking Your Weight

As soon as you begin the keto diet, you must begin tracking your weight. Weigh yourself regularly, and also track body fat and waist circumference.

Here is a graph of my own journey. As you can see below, the fat came off very fast in the first few months and then stayed off *[FIG 2.9]*.

I used the **Yunmai Smart Scale** (with Bluetooth) to track everything for me daily:

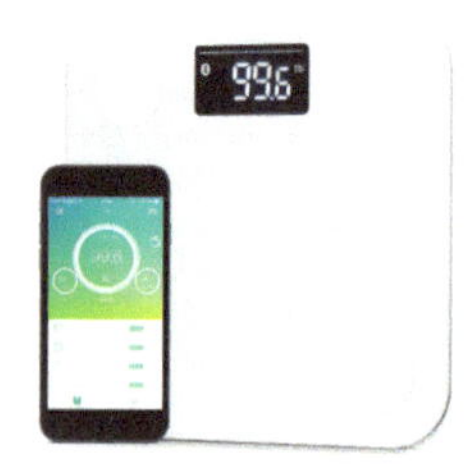

Weight Loss

In the first few weeks on a low carb diet, you may lose 5 to 10 pounds (your cells are letting go of excess water waste being stored in glycogen; for every 1 gram of carbs your cells carry 2 grams of water). After that you should expect to lose about 1 pound a week if you have lots of weight to lose, like I did.

As you continue the diet, you will experience plateaus along the way. Stick with it. It may take 4 weeks or more for you to see your results pick up again. The body has many hormonal cycles and is affected by the time of the year, stress, and all sorts of factors (more on what happens with women's bodies and hormones later). While you want to track your daily data, take a longer-term view. Don't be discouraged if you see a weight gain or plateau one day. Stick with the game plan; the diet will work over time.

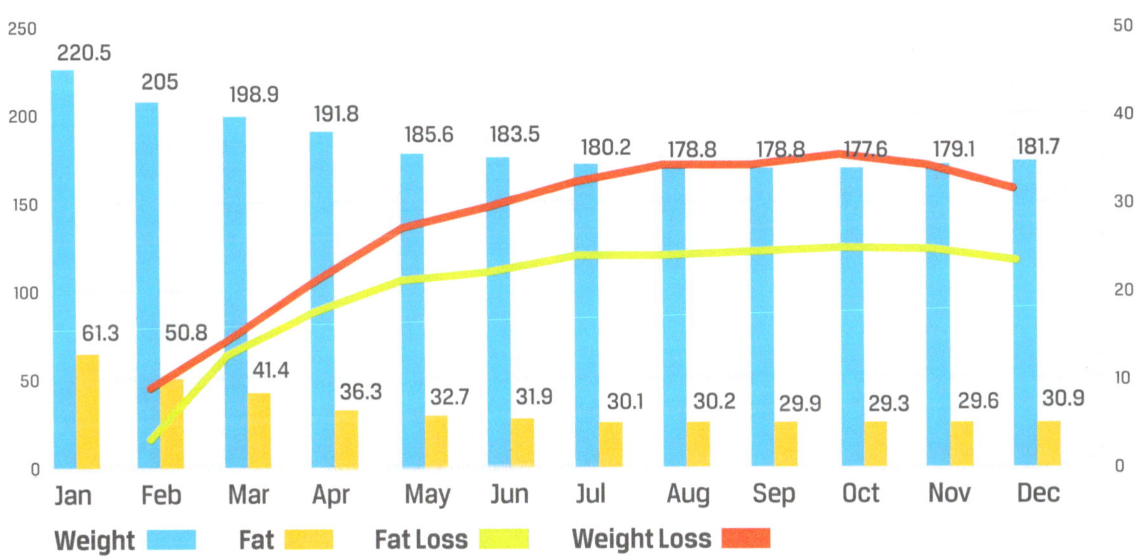

FIG 2.9 ***John's Weight Loss***

Weight Loss Goals

After the first week, set your goal at 1 pound of fat per week. If you do the math, this would be 52 pounds in a year. Every 5 pounds of fat loss should be about an inch lost around the waist. The stricter on low carbs your diet is, the faster you will lose weight. As you get leaner, the weight loss will slow. (Note that women will have a period of time with no weight loss due to the monthly cycle of hormones.)

Take your weight twice a day at the same time every day. I do this first thing in the morning when I am technically in a fasted state, and then in the evening when I get home before dinner. Make sure to track your numbers in some form. For example, I keep an Excel sheet on my hard drive that I've been updating for years.

Weight Loss Stalls and Plateaus

It is not uncommon to see the number on the scale stall. This doesn't mean you are not losing fat. Your overall weight is a combination of muscle, water, fat, and bone. Our water weight fluctuates up and down. Also, the amount of food in the digestive tract goes up and down. Focus in on your waist circumference to see the result of the efforts even if the scale doesn't show it yet.

Many times, people feel like they have hit a plateau when they don't see the daily drop in weight. This is not a plateau. Plateaus are when you have not lost any weight for **4 weeks**. If this happens, then you have hit a real plateau. Start checking your ketone levels and review your macros to get back on track.

Eventually your body will reach a point where further weight loss requires a true lifestyle shift. For me, getting below 16% requires living like a keto bodybuilder. I have experimented with this (more in chapter 6), but it is a totally restrictive and measured lifestyle, requiring specific advice and regimens.

COACHING STORY: Kermit

Kermit was a 65-year-old man who was well over 300 pounds when he started eating keto. He was on high blood pressure medication, statins, and a few other things, just like most American men and women his age.

After learning about the ketogenic diet and fasting, Kermit lost over 100 pounds in eight months.

After the first 30-pound weight loss, he didn't need to be on blood pressure medication anymore. He also went off statins and got rid of his gout.

Kermit was disciplined about what he ate, but the biggest way his diet changed wast that he skipped a lot of meals. He just wasn't as hungry anymore.

But he isn't lower in energy, which isn't surprising considering it is difficult to be over 300 pounds and highly energetic. He reports high levels of energy and he loves the food you can eat on a keto diet.

He wasn't an inactive guy before. He would play golf three times a week and walk all 18 holes. Kermit probably did more of a cardiovascular workout than I did, considering his weight.

One of Kermit's biggest problems before was his huge beer belly. He carried a lot of his weight there. He had assumed eating a keto diet would mean giving up beer, but that isn't true. Now he just drinks low carb instead—and doesn't have that Snickers before bedtime.

Low carb beers are below 3 grams of carbohydrates. I know a lot of guys who like having their beer (me included), so a nice weekend meal for me is a steak and 5-6 beers. That can still work on the keto diet, it's just a matter of tracking what you eat and understanding your macros.

(*Sidenote*: a buddy and I did a "No Drink November" challenge one year while also eating keto. Interestingly, while it was good to have no alcohol, we didn't see any additional weight loss. In my buddy's case, it was because he just replaced the beer with another, equally unhealthy food: we all have our comfort foods and behaviors. In my case, it was because I didn't stick to it. The real lesson? **When things become too mentally tough, they're not sustainable.**)

Remember, it's not no-carb, it's *low*-carb. While not all carbs are equal, you can experiment and still stay in those numbers to get the basic effect of eating a keto diet.

Habit Tracking

There are many options for tracking what you're eating, but the most important thing is to make sure you choose one habit tracker and stick with it. I recommend the *myfitnesspal* app. It is free and can track your food and your macros.

In the app, you can set a goal based on your weight. Then, you simply scan the box or food product to register the macros. Many restaurants have uploaded their macros for menu items. Just search and select. It's very easy and reinforces the good habits you are trying to maintain.

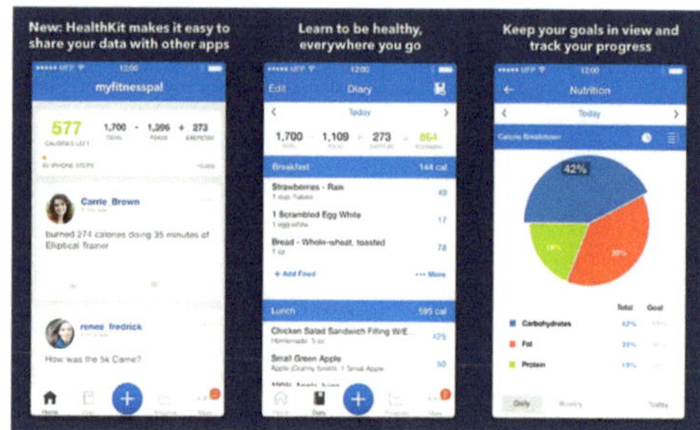

GET STARTED TODAY FREE 14 DAY KETO DIET PLAN

www.dietdoctor.com/low-carb/keto/diet-plan

To Cheat or Not?

I'm asked a lot about whether to cheat on the diet or strictly stick with it. The first thing to understand is being in ketosis is like a light switch; either you are in or you are out.

A study by Dr. Dominic D'Agostino looked at two groups of athletes who were doing resistance training on keto. One group did strict ketogenic dieting 7 days a week; the other did 5 days of strict ketogenic dieting during week and ate carbs on the weekend.[20]

What he found was both groups lost weight and gained muscle. The group that only did 5 days of ketogenic dieting only entered into ketosis after 4 days on the diet, meaning they only got one day of benefit from ketosis a week. They had a lot less fat loss.

Cheat meals can kick you out of ketosis for many days after a high carbohydrate meal. It will be easier to get back into ketosis the longer you have been fat adapted, but you pay a price. So, unlike other diets, you can't do it partially.

With that being said, I do encourage you to have a cheat meal now and then. Plan to do it around celebrations like birthdays or holidays. Have some cake, pizza, and whatever else you want. You should not miss out on life. Yes, you will be kicked out for a few days. But it's not the end of

20 https://dominicdagostino.wordpress.com/2016/06/17/how-the-ketogenic-diet-helps-athletes/

KETO AND TRAVEL

To be a road warrior and follow a ketogenic diet, you have to be prepared. Here's the first thing to know: travel is stressful. When most people travel, their cortisol levels rise, which in turn makes you hungry.

I have tried intermittent fasting while traveling (we delve into this in the next chapter), but it didn't work for me. I am always effing starving by the time I am on the airplane and there are way too many temptations. Remember, elevated cortisol levels make you ready to run from a tiger. When you travel, this is where your mind is at – survive, survive, survive.

So, fasting is out – but you can still stick to keto. Just be prepared. First, always have a bag of macadamia nuts with you. When you get on the airplane and realize you're stuck and hungry, the first thing the flight attendant hands you will be a bag of carbs (i.e. pretzels or snack mix). Even if they are giving you peanuts, the carb count of those is still too high because they will be covered in seasoning, preservative, etc.

Second, make sure you have something to drink. I usually haul single servings of Ultima Replenisher with me and four to five servings of Pique Tea, a fasting green tea. I will also drink coffee black. You can use half and half – but beware: this has a higher carb count.

In terms of heavier snacks, I am a huge fan of FBOMB, especially the chocolate macadamia nut flavor with MCT oil. These are more on the sports nutrition side and have 250 grams of fat. FBOMB also makes cheddar sticks and various other kinds of nut butters that are pre-made in packets and have 250-300 grams of fat. I also like beef sticks from Country Archer. They are nitrate-free and easy to carry.

Another brand I'll stock up on is Good Fats bars. These are lightly sweetened with stevia and come in a variety of flavors. I like the chocolate peanut butter ones personally. Just one of these will keep you full for hours. Perfect Keto makes an almond butter brownie that is great, too. They have 9 grams of protein and 6 grams of fiber.

the world and you won't regain a ton of weight from a day or two. Besides, it's good for you emotionally to have the things that you are missing. It will make your discipline that much easier during your weeks in ketosis.

If you have successfully committed to the keto diet, I would recommend one cheat meal a month. You will likely be back in ketosis the next day if the meal is 150 carbs or lower. I wouldn't do it more frequently than every 3 weeks if you are still trying to lose weight. At the very least, be very strict for the first two weeks you are eating keto. There isn't much room for error there as your body is learning to adjust.

I recently did the ultimate experiment to see what would happen if I went back to my old eating habits. I went on a seven-day cruise, eating everything in sight. My starting weight pre-cruise with my glycogen fully depleted from continuous ketosis was 184.6 lb. I ate double entrées, lots of bread, desserts full of sugar, sugar drinks, and topped it all off with late night pizza and sandwiches. Probably six meals a day. After returning I had Jack-in-the-Box, with the bun and fries, followed by Chinese food with fried rice and all.

At the end of my free-for-all of eight days my stomach hurt badly from all the food bloat and water retention of eating high carbohydrates. And, oh boy, did my weight change. I put on 15.9 pounds, so I was now 200.5 pounds. This was my first time in over two years (since March 2017) I was over 200 pounds. I was a little alarmed, to be honest. Maybe I overdid it?

So, starting the following morning I kicked off a fast to see what my real weight was post-cruise without all the bloat I was retaining. The first 12 hours of fasting, I lost 6.9 lbs. Clearly water weight from the excess carbs and food stuck in me. The following morning, I was down to 189.8 lbs. At the end of 48 hours of fasting I was at 186.3 lbs., a little less than 2 pounds from my starting cruise weight. This is my actual weight gain from the most extreme eating I could do in 8 days.

So, long story short, a cheat meal is not going to cause you to gain 10 pounds. You might weigh more the next day from water retention and the restoration of your glycogen, but a few days of keto will return you to your starting weight.

If you are going to have a cheat meal, there is an effective way to do it. Instead of carbo-loading because you believe you are restoring your muscle glycogen (your muscles already have plenty), stay within the ketogenic spectrum, but pump up the calories.

The thinking behind this relies on **three hormones** in our body. Leptin is the hormone that lets us know when we're hungry. If we stay in a ketogenic state for too long, our brain will start ignoring leptin signals, becoming leptin-resistant. Ideally, we need to spike leptin to continue ketosis without flooding our body with the insulin that comes from carbs, repressing glucagon.

So, if we simply have an influx of ketogenic calories that spike our leptin, we then get that spike of glucagon without the accompanying insulin reaction. Experts recommend a 30% increase in calories to effectively do this.[21]

Remember, we humans are designed for feast and fast. Enjoy life and feast now and then. It's

21 https://www.youtube.com/watch?time_continue=353&v=B2YfqA-amu4I

good for you. Just remember to balance it out with some fasting!

Diet Breaks vs. Cheating

There is a big difference between "cheating" on your assigned keto diet and taking a purposeful break from your keto diet. If keto is going well for you and keto is binary (you're either in or you're out), why would you stop eating keto?

The newest research is showing that, because your body becomes adapted to any diet after a period of time, you have to switch it up, keto included. After reading all the cutting-edge science, I decided to experiment with this for myself. I would sometimes plateau but find that no amount of fasting would help me get out of it. So, what did I do? I ate carbs.

Yes, carbs. Eating carbs results in a hormonal reset. They trigger leptin, which signals your body to produce more thyroid to speed up metabolism. Preferably, you use clean carbs, like lentil noodles (not all carbs are equal). This works because when you are in a fasted state, you are in "protect mode." Once you eat, you enter "repair" mode again.

This isn't the last time you will see the idea of a "diet break" in this book. The fancy term being used for it now is "cyclical ketogenic diet." You aren't permanently in ketosis. Instead, you take breaks, which resets your hormones and builds metabolic flexibility.

I will build on this idea more in the next chapter on intermittent fasting. While fasting itself is a powerful tool—the simplest way to be in ketosis—there are nuances. The way that you break a fast, the length of time you fast, and how often you vary your fast will all amplify or detract from the benefits you get from being in ketosis. To see the best results, you have to take breaks and vary your diet plan.

COACHING STORY: Katherine and Don

Katherine and Don are a couple I began coaching who wanted to lose weight for various reasons. I gave them the basic tutorial, and they had a few questions about my own keto habits. They were both shocked to find out that I actually ate carbs.

"Of course, I eat carbs," I told them, "I'm not the keto police!"[22]

Like so many other people, they thought eating a ketogenic diet meant never touching a carb again or risk ruining all the hard work they had done. Most people trying to lose weight cut carbs like they're poison. They think they're never going to eat cake again or enjoy a regular beer.

But this totally misses the point of what keto is about. It's feast and fast, not fast and fast. Keto isn't a no-carb diet; it's a *low*-carb diet. Carbs aren't the enemy forever. It's just counter-productive to have them too frequently.

I decided to totally level with them.

"Actually, I will eat close to 50 grams of carbs post-workout."

They almost fell out of their chairs.

22 The keto police are a big deal in the world of serious keto-heads. Don't read the comments on any lecture or keto recipe testing video is all I'm saying. If it doesn't pass the keto purity test for these guys, watch out!

I don't share that with most people when they begin eating keto because they don't have the same metabolic flexibility that I do. After my workout, my body is able to handle that many carbs and actually stay in ketosis.

For them, the goal is just to get their body into fat-burning mode - and they have to be fairly rigid to do so. For **at least 14 days**, they need to be on top of their macros. It can take some people as many as 7–8 days to get into ketosis and then another week to adjust.

You can't start off with a cyclical diet of 5 days on, 2 days off, but that's okay for maintenance later. If you do slip into a cyclical pattern, it isn't the end of the world and you won't see a massive weight gain. It just isn't getting you to your goals.

What I mostly see is that people take things so literally. Both the people in the comments on keto YouTube videos (what I like to call the "keto wars") and people I coach. The reality is that it is fine to experiment. Find what works best for body and your lifestyle while paying attention to the science and the numbers to create the optimal program for you.

Exercise on Your New Ketogenic Diet

One of the first questions I am asked by anyone I coach is, "Okay, I get the diet, now what about my exercise routine?" Here's what I tell them: You don't need one.

Yes, eventually I will help them fit exercise into their lifestyle. But, if you are someone who is not currently active, making both a dietary and physical activity change at the same time can be too much. Weight loss is **not** about exercise, so it is most important that we get you rolling on the diet, and then we can discuss how to augment that with exercise.

Even when people are ready to start introducing exercise into their regimen, it's going to look totally different than they might expect. Most people who have excess weight to lose are put on harsh training regimens, the kind that even fit people find grueling. This is totally overdoing it. The workouts are too hard on your body, especially if your body has excess weight. Lactic acid buildup can be extremely damaging. The psychological damage of undergoing and hating intense workouts is also no good.

Also, working out is dangerous for someone interested in weight loss. Why? For the simple fact that it increases hunger. Even if you are at the weight you want, most people will do a big workout and then take that as a sign that they can now eat a huge meal. But the two don't correlate. Remember, calories in does not equate with calories out. Most people would be shocked to see how few calories they are actually burning in a workout anyway.

Exercise is just 10% of our healthy lifestyle. Diet is the foundation, and then appropriate rest (for example, sleep) comes next. I can't emphasize enough how critical rest and sleep are. If you don't get your body resting, it never has a chance to repair, and it is in a constant state of stress.

No science says that humans are supposed to be running 50 miles a week. We are totally overtraining ourselves. So, ditch the hour-long cardio classes. They aren't helping you lose weight, and they're too hard on your body. Instead, go for a long walk.

Walking is the preferred method for exercise when you start your ketogenic diet because it encourages the body to use fatty acids for fuel in your muscles. As you become fat adapted, your muscle cells will begin to use fatty acids directly instead of converting them into ketones.

When you begin your walking workouts, the key is that you have to keep your heart rate under 120 or 130 bpm. That's the difference between aerobic versus anaerobic exercise. When your muscles are engaged in fast twitch, high intensity activity, they need glucose to power them; they can't use fatty acids. But, when your heart rate remains low during exercise, you can burn fat directly and your fat oxidation goes up.

The more you train anaerobically, the more aerobic flexibility you develop. For example, professional long-distance runners will go on long low-intensity runs in order to increase their V02 max, or level of fat oxidation, tapping into fat rather than glucose as their primary energy source.

Chapter Conclusion

There you have it. Contained in this chapter is all the information you need to know to get started on the ketogenic diet.

I find that most people are energized by the ideas I lay out here and want to try them. Then they stumble around for a few weeks, testing stuff out for themselves and end up coming back with more questions once they have some familiarity.

Don't worry if you haven't retained all the information in this chapter. Make your plan, and then feel free to refer to this chapter frequently as you get some keto experience under your belt (or feel free to check out my website www.theketocoach.com for more handy guides and even personal coaching).

But don't quit reading quite yet. More detailed information on topics like exercise and how women's hormones affect weight loss follow. And the most important topic is still to come: intermittent fasting. Intermittent fasting will be one of your most powerful weight loss tools. When I discovered it, it changed my life. Read on for how to combine a ketogenic diet with intermittent fasting to get totally in tune with your body's needs.

The Ketogenic Diet and Athletes

If you are an athlete or a former athlete, you probably have a lot of questions. Working out is bad for me? It can be, especially how amateur athletes approach it. My bet is you have spent your whole life overtraining.

If you are an athlete, I highly recommend you read Charlotte Campbell's The Ketogenic Diet for Athletes. She debunks many popular exercise myths and gives wonderful keto tips for active people. Most notably, she describes how eating a keto diet can improve athletic performance. Once you shift from being a glucose-dependent machine, your V02 maxes improve 15-20% and your peak performance window broadens. Keto athletes are in much less danger of "bonking" and hitting a blood sugar low.

So cut those weird sugary gel and goop supplements from your diet and get smart about your training. Campbell describes decreasing athlete's overloaded workout regimens and getting people to just... walk. Guess what? Their performance was enhanced.

I can speak to this personally. I was curious about how eating a keto diet had affected my own ability to work out and utilize my fat stores. I put this to the test over a day of snowboarding in Colorado.

And speaking of hormones, you can get those endorphin highs from short burst weightlifting and HIIT classes just as easily. No need to spend ninety minutes on the treadmill. Don't train hard; train smart.

INTERMITTENT FASTING + LCHF FOR FASTER RESULTS

Beyond eating a ketogenic diet, the best tool you can have in your arsenal is—fasting.

Fasting is widely misunderstood in our culture today, but it is a universal and historic practice. It has been employed across religions and cultures to do everything from enhance spiritual experiences to promoting mental clarity to controlling weight.

The actual definition of fasting? It is simply the period between the times you are eating. The body technically fasts every night from your last meal, typically dinner, until you eat in the morning. Think about it: the word "breakfast" means "to break your fast." We naturally fast every night while we sleep. The body is designed to be able use stored energy over night to regulate our blood sugar so we don't have to wake up to eat every few hours.

Fasting is an evolutionary function. The body evolved to be able to switch between fuel sources to accommodate the changing food environment.[23] For most of human evolution, we would experience periods of little to no food during which the body relied on stored food fat to provide the needed energy to survive. "Winter" is another name for the period that could last months for our ancestors where they lived mostly on body fat. In modern times, we rarely miss a single meal and almost never go a full day without eating.

Intermittent fasting is the process of extending the overnight fast or the period between eating. If you were to skip breakfast and not eat till lunch, you would extend your fast from 12 hours to 18 hours.

Why would you do this? After all, most of us have been told that it's important to continually snack to keep your metabolism raised.

Not true. There is no medical science that indicates that snacking revs your metabolism. But there is plenty of medical proof that eating does exactly one thing: raise your insulin levels.

So, the benefit of fasting is that you are lowering insulin level by not eating. Your insulin will stay elevated for around 12 hours after a meal.[24] If you don't eat, those levels come down.

23 https://www.cambridge.org/za/academic/subjects/life-sciences/ecology-and-conservation/adaptive-herbivore-ecology-resources-populations-variable-environments?format=PB

24 https://www.hsph.harvard.edu/nutritionsource/carbohydrates/carbohydrates-and-blood-sugar/

The longest medically supervised fast was 382 days without food.[25] The study was conducted by a Scottish university medical team. The twenty-seven-year-old male subject started at 456 pounds and ended the fast at 180 pounds. He lost *276 pounds*. Five years after the fast, the man's weight was constantly around 196 pounds. He experienced no medical problems during or after this fast. He ate no solid food and only took a vitamin supplement along with potassium/sodium supplements.

During the first four months of his fast, the man had a blood sugar reading of 30 mg/dL. In the later months, his reading dropped to 20 mg/dL, which is normally regarded as hypoglycemia territory. But the man did not experience any symptom of hypoglycemia.

I know this story so well—I can write every detail above without looking at my notes—because it was constantly in my mind as I did my first fast. In fact, fasting was my introduction to eating keto. I had read *Tools of Titans* and hopped onto dietdoctor.com. I decided I should do a three-day fast to jumpstart my body into ketosis.

That's right: a three-day fast. I had no idea what to expect. Which is good, because it was *terrible*.

I had every symptom of the keto flu and no clue what to do about it. I had no idea about the need for salt. I had never thought about taking supplements. The only reason I didn't immediately break the fast was that I would think about that guy in Scotland. If he could last 382 days, I at least knew I wasn't going to die.

I still have no idea how I did it, other than sheer will power.

From then on, fasting was something I experimented with on and off. I still didn't have

25 https://www.ncbi.nlm.nih.gov/pmc/articles/PMC2495396/

the proper tools. My staff always knew when I was fasting, because I would be in a terrible, grumpy mood. It didn't click for me until I finally got fed up and got a blood meter. With the blood meter, I had 100% clarity into whether my body was in ketosis or not.

The kicker was that, because of how I was sometimes mismanaging my salt and fluid intake, sometimes I was fasting and not even in ketosis! Clearly, I had a lot more to learn. So, I went back to the books, the lectures, and the online resources. I learned everything I could. I was fascinated.

One important note is that there is a difference between *starving* and *fasting*. In starvation mode, your body will break down all kinds of stuff to in order to feed itself, including muscle. But, if you have gone through keto adaptation, your body is not starving. It has the ability to access its fat stores and keep you healthy while fasting.

COACHING STORY: John the Football Player

John is an active semi-pro football player who works for me. He is well over 300 pounds and carries a huge amount of both muscle and fat.

In the off season, I helped coach him to get down into the high 290s; he doesn't like being at his playing weight all year because it's a lot of stress on his body. Then, he bulks back up when his season rolls back around. I'm not talking about 10 or 20 pounds. John is intentionally yo-yoing 100 lbs every six months or so.

John trains year-round; he gets up at 3:00 a.m. to work out. He is a super disciplined guy. If his exercise and fitness level don't change, what causes the weight fluctuation? His diet. Pre-season, he eats a lot of carbs to bulk up, according to a diet plan his coach has given him. He gets close to 400 pounds.

Then in the off season, he goes on a ketogenic diet. He came to me this year because he had been doing pure keto and had plateaued. I had him add intermittent fasting.

He just does a simple intermittent fast: 16/8. He eats during an eight-hour window. That was enough for him to start to take weight off again. He is now at 260 pounds down from 380 during the season.

Fasting to Repair Your Body

Fasting for me is not just about weight loss; it's about healing. Fasts exceeding 24 hours are *massively* healing to the body. Fasting blood sugars will drop everyday as the body uses up glycogen stores. My normal fasting blood sugar after an overnight fast of 12 hours is around 100 to 110 mg/dL. Two days into a fast, my blood sugar will drop to 70 mg/dL. In four days' time, that number can be below 50 mg/dL.

During longer fasts, people may experience coldness and headaches. Coldness is caused by the lack of blood sugar in the blood stream and not high enough ketone levels to make up for this. This is a temporary state that usually only lasts a day or two. When your ketones get above 1.5, you will feel full of energy and warm again.

The headaches are usually caused by lack of electrolytes. Take a tablespoon of salt in water and the headache should go away in thirty minutes. Just like when you begin eating a ketogenic diet, when you fast the body gets rid of excess water that it had stored from eating carbohydrates. When you lose this water, you also lose salt.

One of the main causes of metabolic syndrome is fat accumulation on the liver and pancreas. The organs will only use this fat up when there is no food in the blood, i.e. in a fasted state. Diet expert Dr. Jason Fung uses three 24-hour fasts a week combined with an LCHF diet at his clinic in Canada to completely reverse type-2 diabetes over three weeks of treatment.[26] (I highly recommend checking out his work; you'll be stunned and encouraged by the results.) He also has two books out, *The Complete Guide to Fasting* and *The Diabetic Code.*

The main reason fasting is healing is that it repairs proper function of the liver and pancreas by causing the accumulated fat to be burned, which lets the organs function properly again. Most of Dr. Fung's patients are able to reduce their medicines and then eventually eliminate them all together.

26 https://www.ncbi.nlm.nih.gov/pmc/articles/PMC6194375/

Intermittent Fasting

Many medical experts with experience in the field now recommend intermittent fasting (IF), versus prolonged fasting, as shown by the science above. That would mean one day of regular eating followed by a 16:8 (16 hours of fasting from 8:00 p.m. to noon; 8 hours of eating from noon to 8:00 p.m.) —or longer—fast. Then, the following day you eat normally.

Studies have shown a larger weight loss for people who do intermittent fasting for two weeks and then take a two-week break, versus doing 4 weeks straight of IF.[27] This allows your metabolism to reset to a higher burn rate during the non-fasting weeks. Continued calorie restriction will lead to a slowing of your metabolism.

On the off weeks, we still want to concentrate on keeping our insulin low by keeping our eating window to 12 hours. If your last meal was at 7:00 p.m., you wouldn't eat again until after 7:00 a.m. the following morning.

I have found intermittent fasting to be an incredibly powerful tool. Rather than simply trying to restrict calories, you are just cutting out an entire meal and immediately putting your body into a stressed state (which is good!).

Some people find themselves frustrated with their weight loss on keto. They aren't making as much progress as they would like. Even though they are burning fat, they are still in calorie surplus. Or they have hit a plateau. Fasting is a surefire way to correct both.

But you have to learn to pay attention to your body when you are in a fast. Sometimes, for reasons I can't figure out, fasting doesn't work for me. I'll be twelve hours in and I'm just dragging butt. Like I have run ten miles and don't have anything left in the tank. This is a sign it's time to eat something, thus breaking my fast.

But I have gotten much better at fasting as I have continued to experiment. Below is what I have learned to make fasting a positive and powerful tool, the best way to kickstart your body into ketosis.

COACHING STORY: Sean

When I started coaching Sean, he was 265 pounds. Six months after he started eating a keto diet, he had totally transformed his body.

Sean is a former Navy SEAL and a super competitive guy. I knew that if I told him about my longest fast, he would want to beat it. That's exactly what happened.

Fasting is the best way to jumpstart your body into ketosis, but it's usually hard to get people to agree to try it much less stick it out. By day 9, Sean had lost 14 pounds. It took him a full week to get into ketosis.

He had lost over 3% of his body fat.

And he felt *awful* for that first week. I think the only way he stuck it out it is grit and wanting to beat me. For the next week, he was in a deep state of ketosis, measuring high 3 ketones for many weeks after that.

Sean continued to experiment with fasting in the weeks following. That's how he still eats today. Like me, he goes by OMAD: "one meal a day." He doesn't track his calories. If he feels like he's not losing weight fast enough, he extends his fast. And he doesn't exercise at all.

For his one meal, Sean usually will eat two ribeye steaks, about 2,000 calories, worth of food. We've started talking about leafy greens and salad, but who cares? He's already healing himself by getting his body into ketosis and losing that weight. We're just taking it step by step.

From February to May, Sean lost 40 pounds. Now he wants to get under 200 pounds. That next step will be difficult. We are trying to reduce 20 years of damage to the body.

He has plateaued with OMAD, so now we are trying a different strategy: two 36-hour fasts a week. I know from personal experience and my reading that weight loss happens after 36+ hours. For most people, two 48-hour fasts work well.

When you plateau, it's important you mix it up. Try different fasting ranges especially. Everyone is different, so it can take time to find the optimal range for you. Also, see my section on taking a diet break.

What to Drink or Eat While Fasting

While you are fasting, you are not allowed any solid foods. But you can drink:

* Water
* Water with salt (pink Himalayan salt preferred or Readmans Real Salt)
* Coffee (without sweeteners or creamer)
* Tea (without sweeteners or creamer)
* Apple cider vinegar ginger drink (Bragg's)

You may not have diet soda or anything with artificial sweeteners. While these do not technically break your fast, they do make you hungry because they incur an insulin response. But you should absolutely be consuming some kind of electrolyte.

You can consume some supplements while on your fast, but I don't recommend it. The entire idea behind a fast is to put stress on your body

27 Thomas DeLauer.

ELECTROLYTE REPLENISHER:

The Ultimate Replenisher is my favorite, but ZipFizz is also really nice. It has the highest level of absorbable potassium. This is good for eating days, especially if you are cramping. Powerade 0 is another option, but I am not a huge fan of those sugar replacements. Gatorade has also come out with an option, but it likely has the same issue.

so that it begins healing itself on a cellular level. If you feed your body supplements before it can get into that state, you defeat the purpose of the fast.

Hunger

While you will be hungry on your fast, remember: fasting is not the same thing as starvation. To better distinguish between the two, let me explain a little what your body feeling hunger is actually about.

Ghrelin is the hunger hormone. It is usually lowest in the morning and will peak in the evenings around 7:50 p.m. It comes in waves. When you are fasting and you feel hungry, you should just ride the wave out. It usually goes away in an hour.

To help with hunger pains, drink a cup of hot coffee or tea. The antioxidants in both those drinks alleviate hunger. Hunger pains are very normal while fasting and not a reason to break your fast.

FASTING SIDE EFFECT: Insomnia

One side effect of fasting that I commonly experienced was increased insomnia during longer fasts. This is normal as your body is producing cortisol, the stress hormone, because you are not eating. It is also a sign that you might have heavy metal built up in you.

I spent two months on a special program to facilitate the process of detoxing from heavy metals.

How was it? Effing horrible. I still am not sure if there were any real benefits to the process, but I do know that my body sloughed off some weird stuff.

What actually helped me was the second thing I tried: red light therapy. As soon as I began red light therapy, my insomnia issues disappeared. The first time I did it, I had the best night of sleep I have maybe ever had, and that was 36 hours into a fast. I even got up at 5:00 a.m. and worked out, and I felt great.

The light I purchased for red light therapy is made by a brand called Joovv. Red light therapy is necessary because most of us are no longer outside enough to get enough red light, an important part of the light spectrum. Instead, we are being blasted by blue light, which is emitted by electric lights, like light bulbs and computers.

Red light is important because it stimulates melatonin, which helps you sleep. Too much blue light and not enough red light kicks you out of natural circadian rhythms, deprives you of melatonin, and makes it very hard to sleep.

5 Ways to Enhance Your Fast

* *Take apple cider vinegar; Bragg makes several apple cider drinks in ginger spice and limeade flavors*
* *Do high intensity interval training (HIIT)*
* *Use a sauna*
* *Break your fast with more protein*
* *Pique tea – matcha green fasting tea*

Muscle Loss While Fasting

One of the most common pushbacks I hear to fasting is that a side effect of fasting is muscle loss, therefore it's an unacceptable strategy for anyone who wants to bulk up or retain their tone.

This is flatly untrue. Remember, fasting is not starving. When you are starving, you will lose muscle mass as the body tries to power itself. But, if you have metabolic flexibility, ketosis is muscle-preserving. Why? Ketones are the answer.

Even if you start the fast not in ketosis, you will burn your existing glycogen stores before you ever start breaking down muscle. Then, you will switch into ketosis. You will begin producing ketones once you are in ketosis, which are inherently muscle-preserving.

Professional body builders actually use this strategy now to cut weight while building their muscle tone. Twenty-four hours into a fast, your HGH levels will be 200–300% higher than normal. Your testosterone will be elevated, too, especially if you are male. With your hormone levels elevated, you work out at the end of your fast, then eat large amounts of protein. Your body is primed to take that protein and move into muscle-building mode, because your high levels of hormones trigger protein synthesis.

We used to think you only had an hour after working out to take advantage of these high hormone levels. In fact, protein syntheses stay high for 24 hours and peak 12 hours in. This is why professional body builders use intermittent fasting to both lose weight and gain muscle at the same time—and in a way that is healthy for their body.

Metabolic Rate Slowdown

Your metabolic rate will inevitably slow down when you are in a fast if your body becomes acclimated to it. This is why you should fast intermittently rather than regularly. You should also vary your fasts. You don't want the restricted calorie state to become your new normal, as any prolonged restricted calorie diet would.

So how do you structure your intermittent fasts?

Fasting Plans

There are many different ways you can go about intermittent fasting. How do you know which plan to choose? It depends on why you are fasting.

Are you fasting for weight loss or healing or longevity?

Fasting for weight loss is easy. If you are not losing weight, fast longer!

But if you are fasting for healing (we'll discuss this in depth later), you need 48 to 72 hours minimum to see healing effects.

Are you interested in longevity? Could I ask a more obvious question? The good news is that any form of calorie restriction fasting has been scientifically shown to extend life. Relative to fasting, there is a minimum of 16 hours to qualify.

16:8 FAST

* 16 hours of fasting, 8:00 p.m. to noon
* 8 hours of eating, noon to 8:00 p.m.

20:4 FAST

* 20 hours of fasting, 4:00 p.m. to noon next day
* 4 hours of eating, noon to 4:00 p.m.
    - From expert Thomas DeLauer
    - 12:00 – Mini meal #1: 25 grams of fat, 25 grams of protein
    - 12:30 – Mini meal # 2: 10 grams of fat, 15 grams of protein
    - 1:00 – Big Meal: 50–80 grams of protein, 40–50 grams of fat
    - 3:00 – dessert: 30 grams of protein, 25 grams of fat

24-HOUR FAST

Eat one meal a day, 24 hours of fasting

36-HOUR INTERMITTENT FASTING

Eat all day through dinner. Then don't eat the following day. Your first meal would be breakfast the following day. You would consume all your calories in a 12-hour window. Don't calorie-restrict on eating days as it will result in a slowdown of your BMR. Example:

- Eat Monday thru dinner
- Fast all day Tuesday
- Eat breakfast Wednesday morning and eat lunch and dinner
- Fast all day Thursday
- Eat breakfast Friday morning and eat lunch and dinner
- Eat Saturday and Sunday

42-HOUR INTERMITTENT FASTING

Eat all day through dinner. Then don't eat the following day. First meal would be lunch the following day. You would consume all your calories in an 8-hour window. Don't calorie-restrict on eating days as it will result in a slowdown of your BMR. Example:

- Eat Monday thru dinner
- Fast all day Tuesday
- Eat lunch Wednesday and eat dinner (can be more meals)
- Fast all day Thursday
- Eat lunch Friday and eat dinner (can be more meals)
- Eat Saturday and Sunday

5-2 FAST

Eat 5 days, fast 2 days

3 TO 5 DAY FAST

72 to 120 hours in length. In these longer fasts you will get into deep states of ketosis with ketone level above 3. This is considered the healing range.

7-14 DAY FAST

Dr. Jason Fung in his Intensive Dietary Management Program often starts his severe type-2 diabetes patients on a 7-14 day fast. This allows the body to adjust to fasting much faster than doing short fasts. Longer fasting periods also create more rapid improvement in blood glucose and type-2 diabetes. Often, he doesn't see an improvement in the blood glucose number until day 5 or 6 of the fast, when he can start reducing the medicine the patients have been on. This result would take much longer using shorter fasting periods. He generally limits the fast to less than 14 days to avoid refeeding situations (more on this below).

14 DAYS AND LONGER

Many people fast for 14 day or longer without any problems. Longer fasts should be observed by a medical provider. If you feel bad anywhere along the way, you should break your fast. You will know the difference between slight hunger pains and the kind of discomfort that necessitates breaking a fast. Your body will feel broken down and drained, like you ran a marathon—not just hungry.

The fast I choose depends on what I am trying to achieve. If I'm just going for maintenance, I do 5/2. But, if I kick off that 5/2 fast with a 24-36 hour fast to get right back into ketosis, I find the whole fast to be much easier because I become fat-adapted that much quicker. I'll plan that initial fast for a Monday, starting the week off right to make up for whatever damage I have done over the weekend. One day of fasting will get me into ketosis if I've had a large carb meal that has kicked me out.

That's the great thing about fasting: it balances you out. Fasting is the simplest way to lose weight if used effectively. You won't see many benefits from just light ketosis, but fasting gets you into deep, deep keto.

I believe that one solid day of fasting has the same health benefits of 10 days of strict keto. Incredible amounts of healing happen when you're not eating at all because you're not adding anything inflammatory to the body. You are giving yourself a break. If you can just eat a few clean meals after your fast, this extends the benefits immeasurably. Which brings us to...

Breaking Your Fast

One of the most important elements of fasting is how you break your fast. Our understanding of this has evolved as the science behind fasting has become more specific. I used to think it didn't matter what I fed my body as I came out of a fasted state, but now I know that, because my body is so sensitive at that time, it matters a lot.

Instead of jumping right into a fat-heavy meal, the best move coming out of your fast is to have a meal of lean protein. This triggers an ideal hormone response. The best ways to break a fast are as follows:

* 6 ounces of lean chicken or turkey (breast, not thigh)
* 6 ounces of shellfish (shrimp or another protein high in omega-3's)
* 6 ounces of fish, such as salmon or clean, small fish sardines or mackerel
* Protein shakes using a grass-fed whey protein
* 1 cup of bone broth (Kettle and Fire is a preferred brand)

Have this mini-meal first. Then an hour later, have your 600-700 calorie meal.

One hormone level you need to watch out for is cortisol. If you're in a fasted state, cortisol will promote weight loss. *But* should this change, cortisol will promote fat storage. Because women are more sensitive to cortisol than men, they can lose weight more effectively if they are in a fasted state.

The flipside is that everyone, and women especially, need to make sure to lower their cortisol levels as they are breaking their fast. Your cortisol will be elevated, so here are the best ways to get it down:

* Go for a walk
* Have coffee with salt and cinnamon (the salt serves as electrolytes; the cinnamon triggers a glucose-like response that gets your cells to open up and release cortisol without the calories)

This is why, if you do a weight workout at the end of your fast, you should break your fast in a very specific way. You have depleted all your muscle glycogen (which is different than your liver glycogen). If you slip a small amount of glucose and fructose (10 grams and 30 grams) into your meal, that energy will get absorbed straight into your muscle. This is called a targeted ketogenic diet.

COACHING STORY: Joe

My buddy, Joe, lost 30 pounds while on the ketogenic diet and utilizing intermittent fasting. Joe is over the age of fifty. Science has shown that, the older you are, the more susceptible you are to slowing down your metabolism.

Joe had plateaued. He was intermittent fasting every day, either only eating two meals or doing OMAD—or one meal a day. He still had a bit more weight to lose and didn't know what to do next. Here was my advice for him:

* First, if you are going to diet or fast, you need to add some variation into your schedule. Remember, any pattern you get into, your body will adjust to. You can make sure you don't slip into this by varying the length of your fast—even fasting longer.
* Second, on your non-fasting day, eat all three meals. Have breakfast, lunch, and dinner. This resets your hormones and allows your fasting days to actually have an effect.

Joe implemented these changes. He felt "less disciplined" (not true—he was doing great), but he added variation. And he was back in business!

What to Watch Out For

REFEEDING SYNDROME

Refeeding syndrome was first described in severely malnourished prisoners after World War II.[28] These people were underweight and didn't have much body fat to begin with. This syndrome has also been observed with anorexics and alcoholics. It is very uncommon in patients with normal body fat stores that are well nourished.

The main cause of refeeding syndrome is that electrolytes have been depleted due to malnourishment. Phosphorus is usually the main culprit. When you eat, minerals like phosphorus and magnesium are critical for the synthesis of glycogen, fat, and protein. If the body cannot get enough of those minerals, it will shut down. This could result in damage to the heart and diaphragm. Low magnesium will lead to cramps, confusion, tremors, and, occasionally, seizures.

Take a multi-vitamin on an extended fast to avoid having any issue. Make sure to add electrolytes to your water. For most people with a normal weight, the occurrence of refeeding syndrome is less than 0.5%.

An additional way to make sure you avoid refeeding syndrome—or just shocking your body in general —is moderating how you come off your fast. Don't go straight for the T-bone steak. Break your fast with some bone broth. Then eat a small meal thirty minutes later. After 1 hour, you can eat a normal meal.

28 https://www.ncbi.nlm.nih.gov/pmc/articles/PMC390152/

DETOXIFICATION

During your weight loss journey, you will experience detoxification. As your body processes fat, toxins that were stored in the fat will be processed and excreted. As your gut shrinks, the sludge that is caking the lower intestines will come loose and pass. It is not uncommon to have very loose stools with black sand-like substance coming out of you. This went on for about three weeks for me as I lost my first 30 pounds.

I recommend that you start taking both a probiotic and prebiotic to improve your lower gut bacteria. The sludge build-up plus a poor diet have led to lower absorption of nutrients in the lower gut. These are the same kind of bacteria that are also killed off every time you have to take an oral antibiotic.

AUTOPHAGY

Autophagy is process that begins four days into a fast wherein the body will recycle damaged or broken-down cells. This process is triggered by insulin dropping and glycogen rising. It is becoming better understood, and even recently has been a hot topic in science. On October 3, 2016, the Nobel Assembly at Karolinska Institute awarded the Nobel Prize in Physiology or Medicine to Yoshinori Ohsumi for his discoveries of mechanisms for autophagy.[29]

When cells become stressed, they have a variety of reactions or cell fate decisions: adaptation, repair, recovery, senescence (cell exit), or apoptosis (cell death).[30] It is critical that the body is put under the kind of stress that triggers these reactions. This response is necessary in order to process cells that could be dangerous—even cancerous. New research is suggesting that autophagy might be critical to tumor suppression. [31]

Having old proteins in your system is the cause of two important diseases: Alzheimer's Disease (AD) and cancer. Alzheimer's comes from amyloid beta or Tau protein building up in your brain.[32] The research around this is still developing, but autophagy could represent an interesting opportunity for further treatment.

29 https://www.nobelprize.org/prizes/medicine/2016/press-release/
30 http://genesdev.cshlp.org/content/23/7/784.full.html
31 Mathew et al. 2007a; Levine and Kroemer 2008
32 https://www.dietdoctor.com/renew-body-fasting-autophagy

FASTING:

"First, if you are going to diet or fast, you need to add some variation into your schedule. Remember, any pattern you get into, your body will adjust to. You can make sure you don't slip into this by varying the length of your fast—even fasting longer."

DRY FAST

Dry fasting is more extreme and should only be attempted with a doctor's supervision. It works the same as an intermittent fast or longer fast with one big exception: no fluid intake. As the body gets dehydrated because of the lack of water intake, it goes into a shock mode. This accelerates autophagy to free up fluids in the body.

Next the body breaks down fat at a faster level to get the hydrogen molecules to mix with the air you breath to create water. You got that, right? The body can create its own water. Studies have shown a one-day dry fast burns as much fat as a three-day fast with fluids.

You can go 16 hours or longer on a dry fast. When breaking a dry fast, you need to be very careful not to overdo the water intake. Drink 1 pint of water and then wait an hour before drinking another. Do this over 6 hours before you drink all you want. Limit your salt intake during these first hours. When you eat, eat a bland chicken breast and limit your fat and salt for the first 6 hours of a refeed.

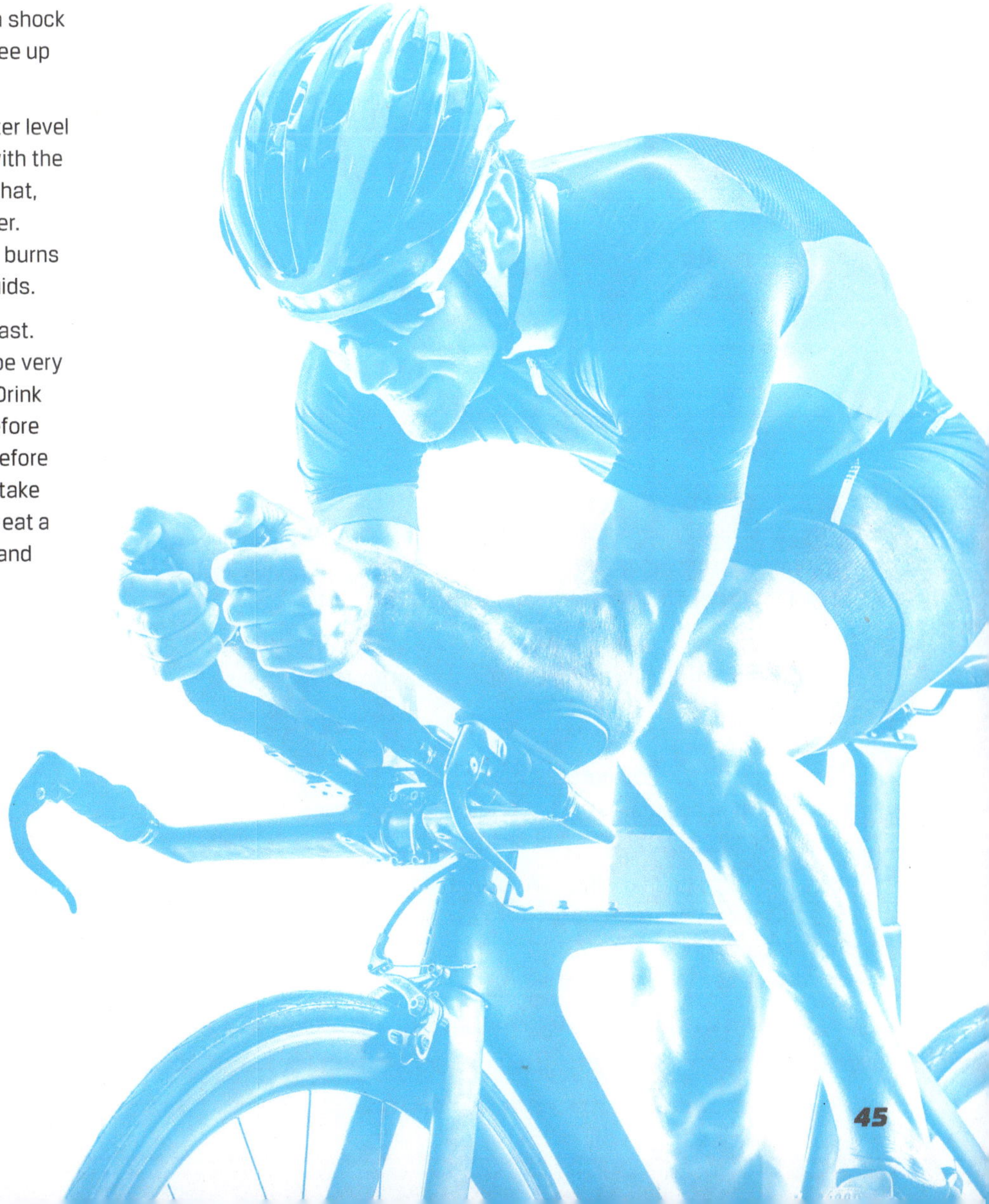

HEALING THE BODY

As I stated in the beginning of the book, a ketogenic diet is not just about weight loss. While eating keto is a handy tool for burning fat and better understanding how your body utilizes energy, it also genuinely promotes a healthier state for your body.

The following conditions can be improved or eliminated by a ketogenic diet combined with intermittent fasting:

* High blood pressure
* Type 2 diabetes
* Heart disease
* Cancer
* Inflammation
* High cholesterol
* Heartburn
* Allergies

In this chapter, I will briefly address each of these conditions, explaining why ketosis is critical in addressing them. I will also direct you to further resources in the event you would like more information.

I know that ketosis plays a key part in improving health because I have seen it in the people I have coached, from my father-in-law to my own daughter.

Knowing Your Cholesterol Numbers

One of the first questions I get from people when I help get them started on the ketogenic diet is: With all that fat, what about my cholesterol?

Cholesterol has traditionally been painted as the "bad guy" that causes heart disease. It has gotten a very bad rap. Here's the thing: when this idea first became popular in the 1960s, there was no science that proved that cholesterol had anything to do with heart disease.

At the time, it was believed that high cholesterol was caused by animal fat. This led to a whole new market of products being pushed that were supposed to substitute for animal fat, like vegetable oil and margarine, to provide a lower saturated fat product. Of course, now we know that those don't lower our cholesterol significantly—and they can cause cancer.[33 34]

Nowadays, the conversation has evolved a little. Rather than just talking about high numbers as a monolith, people often talk about their "good" and "bad" cholesterol. But even this is too simple. Cholesterol is more complicated than just a "good" and a "bad" cholesterol number.

Cholesterol itself is not only not bad, it's critical to how your body functions. It is essentially an **energy transport system**. You will die without it.

Remember that having too high cholesterol was attributed to eating animal fats. If you have been told your cholesterol is high, you will be familiar with the first foods the doctor recommends cutting from your diet: high fats like cream, butter, and red meat. This is not correct. Rather than high fats, highly polished carbs are the culprit.

Triglycerides are caused by carbohydrates, *not animal fat*. VLDL is raised by carbs, not fat. The whole thing was oversimplified to measure total cholesterol because scientists at the time didn't have the equipment to measure the individual factors that actually make up cholesterol. Remember: cholesterol to them was just one number—one number, as it turned out, that represented a whole host of factors.

It was found that high triglycerides were present in heart disease and not cholesterol. The problem

33 https://www.mayoclinic.org/healthy-lifestyle/nutrition-and-healthy-eating/expert-answers/butter-vs-margarine/faq-20058152
34 https://www.dietdoctor.com/low-carb/vegetable-oils

How Cholesterol Became the Bad Guy

Before our food production was industrialized, humans went through natural cycles of feast or fast. Unfortunately, that "fast" could turn to "starve" if nature or other external forces disrupted the food supply.†

As the food supply became steadier, pure calories were more readily available. People were starving less (good!), but new problems started showing up. Mass-produced flour and sugar were a foundational part of people's diets, especially during wartime when most people were put on government rations. We began fortifying our milk, flour, and salt, adding minerals and other critical missing ingredients that we weren't getting in our natural food supply anymore.

Eating an artificially-fortified-but-naturally-deficient diet had one clear impact: an increase in heart disease. Heart disease became public enemy number one. A study was done in the sixties to investigate just why so many people were dying so young of heart disease. The scientists decided that the primary contributing factor was plaque buildup in the heart. And what caused this? Cholesterol. Of course.

If you're nodding your head along like, Isn't that right? It is, but it isn't the whole story. Cholesterol = Plaque = Heart Disease is a gross oversimplification of critical processes to our body's survival. But the result was that cholesterol was treated as one total number in need of suppressing. Drug companies got involved, investing money and resources in coming up with "solutions," marketing those solutions, and then making sure as many people as possible were on those drugs.

† For further discussion, check out Gary Taub's excellent book, *Good Calories Bad Calories*. It's an 800-page tome, but it has everything in there you could want on this subject.

was that triglycerides were very tough to measure as compared to cholesterol. As such, most of the tests focused on just cholesterol in the 1960s. The only way doctors had to measure cholesterol was to put your blood into a centrifuge and spin it out. LDLC—total cholesterol—was the measurement they came up with to describe cholesterol levels, arbitrarily deciding that anything over 200 was bad.

This was a great opportunity for Big Food to pay for study after study showing that fat was bad. Our diets were shaped accordingly. Statins were invented to "lower cholesterol." The rest is history.

Eventually we got a little more sophisticated, moving away from rhetoric and back into science. Cholesterol, we realized is not just LDLC but LDL + HDL, two totally different components. We figured out that high HDL will lower the risk of heart disease. It was and is believed that HDL protects against heart disease, as measured in the 1977 study. The higher the HDL, the lower the LDL & triglycerides.

But LDL itself is broken down into **7 different particles**.

LDL in total is not a predictor of heart disease; only small, dense LDL (Pattern B) causes the blockages. Larger, fluffy LDL (Pattern A) does not oxidize or cause heart disease. It is Pattern B, which is very small LDL, that causes heart disease.

High LDL is a problem. LDL is the end product of VLDL that is produced in the liver, which is a transporter of energy to the cells.

If you want to lower your LDL, you first need to get the liver to stop producing cholesterol. The best way to do this is to stop eating. Start by skipping a few meals here and there and work up to going 24 hours between eating. The body will continue to produce cholesterol as long as it is in a fed state. 70 days of IF can reduce cholesterol by 25%, which is way better than any statins drug.

First you need to know what all your numbers really are, because the composite numbers you have been fed your whole life aren't useful. Tell your doctor that you want the blood test that breaks down the particle sizes of the cholesterol. The test is called NMR 8 panel or NMR lipo subset with lipid clac. Also get your HbA1C measure; this is the real one that predicts heart problems.

* Get your HDL above 50, ideally over 70 (this is the good cholesterol)
* Get your triglycerides below 100, ideally below 50
* Get your LDL below 100, ideally below 70, and have it shift your LDL from small, dense particles to large, fluffy particles. Small particles are caused by carbs and in turn create blockages or plaque. Large-particle LDL is from fat in the diet and does not block the veins.
* Don't worry about total cholesterol. LDL-C is a calculated measurement
* Get an NMR test to see full details
* Get a HSCR test for inflammation and CT scan of the heart

I've implemented the strategies above. Below are what my last results looked like.

The best way to raise your good cholesterol is by eating meat and fat. Remember: 80% of the

3/1/2021 Lab Results

Patient Name: John Hutmacher | **Date of Birth:** 09/04/1977

Note to Patient: The results of your recent lab tests are within normal limits. We look forward to seeing you at your next appointment.

NMR 8 PANEL 03/30/2018 (#1184331, Final, 03/27/2018 8:10am)

Note to Patient: The results of your recent lab tests are within normal limits. We look forward to seeing you at your next appointment.

Report	Result	Ref. Range	Units		Status	Lab
LDL-P	<382	0 - 1299	NMOL/L		Final	COMP
HDL-P	40.5	38.1 - 10000	UMOL/L		Final	COMP
SMALL LDL-P	<152	0 - 749	NMOL/L		Final	COMP
LARGE VLDL-P	2.5	0 - 2.7	NMOL/L		Final	COMP
LARGE HDL-P	14.7	7.4 - 10000	UMOL/L		Final	COMP
LDL SIZE	21.2	20.5 - 10000	NM		Final	COMP
HDL SIZE	10.1	9.2 - 10000	NM		Final	COMP
VLDL SIZE	**49.8**	**0 - 46.6**	**NM**	**IR**	**Final**	**COMP**

LIPIDS/LIPOPROTEINS/APOLIPOPROTEINS

	OPTIMAL RANGE	INTERMEDIATE RISK RANGE	HIGH RISK RANGE	UNITS
LDL-P	<1020	1020-1359	>=1360	NMOL/L
HDL-P	>38.0	34.1-38.0	<=34.0	UMOL/L
sLDL-P	<501	501-1000	>1000	NMOL/L
lVLDL-p	<2.7	2.8-6.9	>6.9	NMOL/L
lHDL-p	>7.3	3.1-7.3	<3.1	UMOL/L
LDL-s	>=20.5			NM
HDL-s	>=9.2	8.9-9.1	<8.9	NM
VLDL-s	<46.6	46.7-52.5	>52.5	NM

TESTING PERFORMED AT COMPASS LABORATORY SERVICES
1910 NONCONNAH BLVD. SUITE 108 MEMPHIS, TN 38132
CLIA NO. 44D2026010

NOTE FROM LAB: PT FASTING

Note: Patients are solely responsible for maintaining the privacy and security of all information print

LIPIDS/LIPOPROTEINS/APOLIPOPROTEINS

	OPTIMAL RANGE	INTERMEDIATE RISK RANGE	HIGH RISK RANGE	UNITS
LDL-P	<1020	1020-1359	>=1360	NMOL/L
HDL-P	>38.0	34.1-38.0	<=34.0	UMOL/L
sLDL-P	<501	501-1000	>1000	NMOL/L
lVLDL-p	<2.7	2.8-6.9	>6.9	NMOL/L
lHDL-p	>7.3	3.1-7.3	<3.1	UMOL/L
LDL-s	>=20.5			NM
HDL-s	>=9.2	8.9-9.1	<8.9	NM
VLDL-s	<46.6	46.7-52.5	>52.5	NM

TESTING PERFORMED AT COMPASS LABORATORY SERVICES
1910 NONCONNAH BLVD. SUITE 108 MEMPHIS, TN 38132
CLIA NO. 44D2026010

cholesterol in the body is made in the liver. The liver produces this **regardless** of what is eaten. The only time it doesn't produce cholesterol is when it is not being fed. In fact, a targeted low-fat diet will actually lead to a drop in the good cholesterol, HDL, and not achieve a reduction in LDL. This is a far bigger problem, according to studies. The better the HDL and LDL *ratio* is, the lower the chance of heart disease.

If you need to reduce cholesterol overall, try fasting to get production down in the liver. If you need to reduce bad cholesterol, you need to stop eating carbohydrates, not fat.

For more information, my favorite book on this subject is *Cholesterol Clarity* by Jimmy Moore. I have given you the basics, but if you want to be a true cholesterol expert, his work is incredibly informative.

Statins are Poison

In the mid 1990s Pfizer Pharmaceuticals introduced the cholesterol-lowering drug Lipitor. It was a hit and is the **most profitable and bestselling drug ever**. [35]

Here's the thing: we only have a *7% chance* of getting heart disease if we are eating as our bodies are meant to. Guess how much statins actually lower our chance of heart disease? **1%**.

That's right. All those cholesterol-lowering drugs that doctors have been pushing on you actually do squat for increasing your heart health. I don't mean to sound anti-doctor—I'm not—but I am against putting drugs in your body for no purpose and to your detriment.

Getting off the statins is crucial so that you can allow your body to operate as it was meant to. As always, consult your doctor before making changes. But explain that you want to try handling your cholesterol in a healthier way. The tools are before you.

Cholesterol Rise on Keto

When you first go on a ketogenic diet it is common for your cholesterol to rise. Your body is releasing stored fat back into the blood stream to be used as fuel. When your weight loss slows, you will see your cholesterol levels return to normal.

35 https://www.businessinsider.com/lipitor-the-best-selling-drug-in-the-history-of-pharmaceuticals-2011-12

Adult Health Examination Tests

- *2830 | Testosterone*
- *2835 | TSH*
- *9179 | Comprehensive Metabolic Pa*
- *1000 | CBC w/auto diff*
- *5083 | High Sensitivity CRP*
- *4288 | Homocystenie*
- *2760 | Insulin*
- *4359 | Lipoprotein A*
- *4004 | Apolipoprotein A-1*
- *4003 | Apolipoprotein B-100*
- *3800 | Blood Group (ABO) and Rh T*
- *4363 | NMR Lipo Subset with Lipid Calc*
- *2708 | Hemoglobin A1C*

Above are some additional tests you may want your doctor to run to get deeper insight into what's going on inside you.

High Blood Pressure

High blood pressure is typically a result of your body holding too much fluid. The modern approach has been to tell patients to limit their salt intake because the kidneys will hold extra water to store that salt.

When cutting salt doesn't work to lower the blood pressure, the doctor will prescribe blood pressure lowering medicine and diuretics to get the fluid out. The medicine will cause the fluid to leave—along with all of your minerals. Next you have to take a huge potassium pill... and on it goes from there.

Salt has been made out to be the enemy. In fact, as always, the real culprit is carbohydrates. For every 1 gram of carbs your body stores, 4 grams of water are stored with it. In addition, most of the low-fat processed foods are filled with salt to make them taste good once they remove the fat.

By going on a ketogenic diet, less than 20 carbs a day will cause the body to naturally shed the stored water and salt. Many people will lose 10 pounds of water weight in the first two weeks once they get into ketosis. This alone is usually enough to start cutting back on the medicine, as now your blood pressure will be too low.

As the stored salt and water get released and your excess weight comes off, your blood pressure will continue to go down.

Type 2 Diabetes

Type 2 diabetes occurs when your body is making too much insulin, often because it has become insulin-resistant. Because keto at its core is about understanding and regulating the hormones that affect weight, keto is an excellent tool in managing type 2 diabetes.

First, make sure to consult with your doctor if you have type 2 diabetes and you are interested in trying a keto diet. There is always a period of adjustment into ketosis, and it is critical that your insulin levels are kept stable during this time.

However, if carefully managed, keto can naturally help regulate those spikes and swings in insulin that medications are artificially managing. Many people either reduce or entirely stop their medications once they are fully adapted to a ketogenic diet.

For more information, read Dr. Jason Fung's book, *The Diabetic Code*.

COACHING STORY: Jennifer

Jennifer was pre-diabetic and then became a type-2 diabetic while I knew her. She was getting prescribed more and more medicine to help manage her diabetes, culminating in a recommendation to go on insulin. Her fasting insulin was more than 120.

Jennifer finally hit a point of frustration. I had given her a great book, *The Diabetic Code*, and I hoped she would read it. I talked with her about fasting and the work that Dr. Fung was doing with his patients. She gave me excuses, telling me she couldn't mess around with any of that stuff because she was diabetic.

I hear that a lot. "I take medicine every day, so I can't do a keto diet."

Usually I just agree and then give the person my "Coaching" document. If they want to try, the information and tools are there for them.

A few weeks went by. Things weren't going well for Jennifer. She had finally had enough.

"You need to cut the sugar with the goal of going back to your doctor and getting off the medicines," I told her. With the consent of her doctor, she agreed.

Keto is a pretty easy diet to get people into. You give them the food guides and explain what is going to be a problem to eat.

Jennifer never really did the fasting, but she did totally change her diet. She was kind of lazy about keto. She never downloaded MyFitnessPal or tracked what she ate. The only tool she had was taking her blood, which, as a diabetic, she was already doing to measure her blood sugar.

For Jennifer, it was just a matter of explaining what she should eat and what she shouldn't eat. That's all she needed to move forward. Just those simple visual guides. Here's what your body wants. Here's what you should stay away from.

And it worked. After adjusting to a ketogenic diet, the results were fantastic. Her fasting blood sugar was below 120 in the morning. She was off her medicines. As a bonus, she had lost 20 pounds.

Type 1 Diabetes

Type 1 diabetes occurs when your pancreas flat out stops producing insulin. People who have Type 1 diabetes must inject themselves with insulin. They usually discover this condition when they are very young (it is an uncommon disease; only 5% of the population has this). The only treatment is a lifelong management of their insulin levels via injection.

The core cause is not treatable with a keto diet, but eating a keto diet can help you manage your insulin levels. However, because having the right insulin levels is so critical to someone with type 1 diabetes, make sure to work with your doctor if you are going to experiment with the keto diet.

Heartburn

Heartburn is caused by acid reflux. Millions of people suffer from it. Many people take very powerful medicine to combat it. This has now been shown to kill off the bacteria in the lower intestine.

Diet can fix heartburn and its core cause, acid reflux. Along my journey, one of my employees started eating keto, too. One of the first things he noticed was that his acid reflux was gone. I became curious about why this had happened and found a study out of Europe that proved the sugar and carbohydrates were causing the GERD (gastro-oesophageal reflux disease).[36] After 10 weeks on a high fat, low carbohydrate diet, all of the patients no longer had GERD and were off their medicine.

36 https://onlinelibrary.wiley.com/doi/full/10.1111/apt.13784

Cancer

This is a complicated topic, but I want to cover it quickly. High level: cancer cells have 10x the amount of glucose and insulin receptors as a regular cell. This is why fasting works so well to attack them. They can't run on fat like the rest of your body. You can starve them to death by fasting or eating a ketogenic diet.

Cancer cells thrive on sugar. In addition, high levels of insulin cause high levels of IGLF, which protects cancer cells from getting killed in regular autophagy.

Clearly, medical treatment is required for cancer, but having a good diet can help your results. For example, fasting before chemotherapy can make chemotherapy more effective at killing cancer cells.

www.youtube.com/watch?v=WnK1FgxflWM

In Thomas Seyfried's book, *Cancer as a Metabolic Disease*, he describes doing a seven-day fast to drive blood sugar low enough to enter a therapeutic range to shrink tumors, since they live on sugar. Dr. Seyfried recommends only having water—no vitamins or anything else—as doing so may be sending mixed signals to the body. In addition, water fasting the day before chemotherapy and the day of chemotherapy have been shown to reduce the effect of chemotherapy on the body and amplify its effects on the cancer cells.

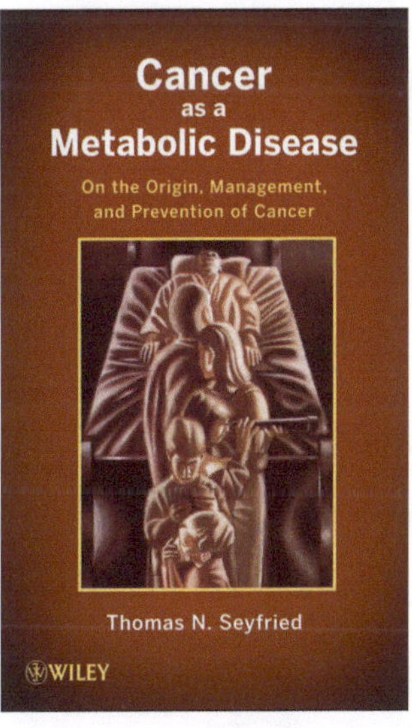

Inflammation

This is one of the most important topics to cover, but I have saved it for proper context. When we're talking about the cellular healing and damage happening in your body via a poor diet, what we are really talking about is inflammation.

Inflammation is simply how your body naturally reacts when it is out of whack, either when it is injured or dealing with a chronic disorder. Your cells signal something is awry, and your immune system kicks in, sending white blood cells and other agents to defend and repair.

But, constantly being in a state of attack is bad for your body. Our modern diet has us almost constantly in a state of inflammation, fighting off the bad toxins that we put in our bodies on a daily basis. Reducing inflammation is a core principle of keto, because inflammation can lead to so many other complicated side effects.

In addition to eating keto, it is important to understand what is going on when you process food so you can continue to refine your diet. Which brings us to...

The Gut

Recent studies have identified how bacteria in the gut are signaling the brain and controlling the immune system in a way that is incredibly damaging.

Lectins are the highest source of inflammation in our diets. They are proteins from certain plant families that target and bind carbohydrates. The body has an incredibly hard time digesting them. They cause damage in our gut that causes harmful toxins to leak into the bloodstream.

A small amount of plant lectins will cause minimal inflammation (as long as you are not a person who is overly sensitive to them), but lectins are toxic to us at the levels we eat today. A great book on the subject is the *Plant Paradox* by Dr. Gundry. He has helped many people fix their diets with a three-phase approach to heal the gut and improve health.

The first two phases eliminate all the lectins from the diet. In phase three, you slowly re-introduce some of them and see if they trigger a return of your inflammation. He explains that gut health is more about what you cut out of your diet versus what you add into it, as in any classic elimination diet.

FOODS TO AVOID OR LIMIT:

* Grains, especially whole grain products
* Grain fed animal products including milk and cheese
* All legumes including peanuts
* Cashews, pine nuts and almonds
* Tomatoes
* Bell peppers
* Seeds
* Cucumbers
* Squash
* Artificial sweeteners and sugar

INFLAMMATION:

"I began my own journey with this several years ago. It was less a diet change, and more a lifestyle change. Once I realized that inflammation is at the root of so much disease and weight gain, I wanted to do my best to reduce inflammation in my own body."

FOODS YOU CAN EAT:

* Grass-fed animal foods
* Wild-caught seafood
* Coconut, macadamia, pecans, pistachios & walnuts
* Coffee
* Dark chocolate
* Olive oil, Avocado oil, coconut oil
* Stevia/ Xylitol / erthritol, monk fruit, yacon, artichoke syrup
* Limit intake of blueberries, raspberries. and strawberries

The basic rule is that you want to avoid any plant that has seeds, like tomatoes, bell peppers, zucchini, cucumbers, and peas. These are all truly fruits and contain vegetable proteins called lectin. Gluten is only one of a thousand lectins.[37]

Legumes like peanuts are also lectins and about 5% of people have a very serious allergic reaction to it because they don't have the enzymes to digest legumes.

A very important note about fruit: all fruit has fructose, which will make you fat if you eat too much of it (we covered this in chapter 2). In addition, store-bought fruit has not ripened naturally and contains very high levels of lectin.

This fruit has been exposed to acetylene gas once it gets to the store, which changes the color of the outside of the fruit, but the lectin on the inside has not been removed by the ripening process. It looks ripe, but it isn't.

His rule is: only eat locally grown fruit at harvest time. Make sure it's organic as well to avoid pesticides.

If you are going to eat carbs, make sure it is white bread made from yeast. Sourdough is even better.

Gluten is one example of a plant lectin that everyone is familiar with. Did you know that many of the gluten-free foods we are eating have even more potent lectins in them than gluten? The worst lectin is WGA, which comes from the bran in whole grain foods and products.

37 https://www.authoritydiet.com/what-lectin-foods-high-lectins/

In addition to lectins, Dr. Gundry lists "7 Deadly Disruptors" to avoid:

1. Broad-spectrum antibiotics
2. Non-steroidal anti-inflammatory drugs
3. Stomach-acid blockers
4. Artificial sweeteners
5. Endocrine disruptors
6. Genetically modified foods (GMO's) and the herbicide Roundup
7. Constant exposure to blue light

We will dive into each of these categories in detail, but here's some simple steps you can take now to start combatting inflammation:

* Take a prebiotic to speed up the rebuilding of your good bacteria.
* Antibiotics and Stevia wipe out your good bacteria and can take two years to rebuild after one batch. Use them wisely.
* Many animals are fed antibiotics, so eating meat is like taking a low-dose antibiotic (unless you're very careful where your meat is coming from).
* Also, grain-fed animals will have higher level of lectin than grass-fed animals.
* Bad gut bacteria crave sugar and can trigger the brain into wanting lots of it.

I began my own journey with this several years ago. It was less a diet change, and more a lifestyle change. Once I realized that inflammation is at the root of so much disease and weight gain, I wanted to do my best to reduce inflammation in my own body.

We had a personal reason for this in our family, too. My daughter has had severe eczema on her hands ever since she was a baby. We tried everything: creams, allergy drops, and every traditional medicinal approach. None of it made any difference.

After we read *Plant Paradox*, we implemented some dietary changes. Boom. We had our answer. Using the elimination diet, we discovered that she had three triggers:

* Tomatoes (which are a nightshade)
* Cucumbers (also a nightshade)
* Wheat (which is a glutinous plant lectin)

As soon as we changed her diet, the eczema cleared up. But, if she eats any one of those three things, it flares back up. Which is a bummer, because her favorite meal is Panera mac and cheese—100% on the no-fly list.

Remember how I said fasting is healing? That's because you aren't triggering any inflammation in the body. Your body can finally calm down. When that had such positive results, I began looking deeper at what was causing inflammation in my lifestyle and routine. I changed my deodorant, my toothpaste, the plastic food storage containers in my kitchen. I began asking myself:

* What are the sources of inflammation in my lifestyle, including my diet?
* How can I eliminate as many sources as possible?

Broad-Spectrum Antibiotics

Over the last 60 years, we have devolved broad-spectrum antibiotics that kill multiple strains of bacteria simultaneously and which have saved many lives. The downside of these is they also kill the good bacteria in our gut that help us break down food and protect our gut lining from plant lectins. It can take up to two years for the good microbes to regrow, and many strains may be gone forever. Every dose a child takes increases the likelihood of them developing Crohn's disease, diabetes, obesity, or asthma later in life.

It not just the prescription from your doctor either. It's in our food. Most of American chicken or beef contains enough antibiotics to kill bacteria in a petri dish.

First, change out your meat to organic, grass-feed beef and pastured chicken to ensure you aren't ingesting antibiotics at every meal. Also, don't take antibiotics when you know it's a virus. If you do have to take antibiotics to get over something, you must rebuild your gut bacteria with pre- and pro-biotics.

Nonsteroidal Anti-Inflammatory Drugs (NSAIDs)

Ibuprofen (Advil and Motrin), Naproxen (Aleve), Celebrex, Mobic, and other nonsteroidal anti-inflammatory drugs have been around since the 1970s and were introduced as an alternative to aspirin. They were introduced because aspirin was known to damage the stomach lining. We now know that NSAIDs damage the mucosal barrier in the small intestine and colon, which allows lectins and other substances to pass through the intestinal wall into the body, triggering inflammation.

Stomach-Acid Blockers

Acid-blocking drugs such as Zantac, Prilosec, Nexium, and Protonix should be avoided at all costs. These drugs reduce the amount of stomach acid. The stomach acid is needed to kill bad bacteria that you swallow. This allows bad bacteria to grow in the small intestine, causing the condition of leaky gut.

If you reduce your carb intake, you will find the acid reflux goes away. Rolaids are a good substitute.

Artificial Sweeteners

A Duke study showed that one packet of Splenda kills 50% of normal gut bacteria. Most artificial sweeteners like sucralose, saccharin, or aspartames will alter your gut bacteria. For most of our evolution, sweet tastes were only available in the summertime from ripe fruit. This taste signaled the body to store fat for winter. We now have sweet tastes available year-round, triggering our body to think it should ramp up storage of fat for winter. Even though these drinks and foods are low-calorie, it triggers you to gain weight as the body is constantly hungry. Stevia, monk fruit, and sugar alcohols like xylitol or erythritol are acceptable replacements.

Endocrine Disruptors

Endocrine disruptors are hormone disruptors that look like estrogen in the body. They come from chemicals found in plastics, cosmetics, preservatives, insecticides, sunscreens, and many daily products. Exposure to these will wreak havoc with your hormones and leads to problems like obesity, diabetes, reproductive issues, cancers, thyroid problems, and autoimmune diseases.

You can find approved products at *EWG.org*.

Genetically Modified Foods (GMOs) and the Herbicide Roundup

Herbicides, insecticides, and pesticides have reduced mosquito diseases and increased crop yields to help feed the world. They have also had the unintended consequence of introducing poisons into our body through the food we eat. Roundup, as an example, kills off critical gut bacteria that are responsible for creating crucial amino acids for the body that produce serotonin, tyrosine, and phenylalanine, required for thyroid production. Many depression and thyroid problems are most likely caused by the food we are eating that is covered in Roundup.

To avoid poising the body, avoid any plants that are not labeled organic, as they were likely sprayed with Roundup. In addition, avoid normal beef, pork, and chicken as they have been fed grain and soybeans that were GMOs sprayed with Roundup. You want to buy grass-fed, grass-finished beef, heritage pork, and pastured chicken. You are what the animals you eat, eat.

Constant Exposure to Blue Light

For thousands of years, animals and humans have responded to the length of day in their eating habits. Long days and short nights signal the body to store fat in preparation for winter while food is still plentiful. Short days and long nights signaled us to look for less food and burn fat. This is mainly triggered by the blue light wavelength from sunlight, triggering a seasonal cycle of hormones to store or burn fat. The problem is that today we are in summer mode year-round due to huge amounts of blue light that we are exposed to from office lights, TVs, cell phones, and other devices, 365 days a year.

The solution is to change your cell phone to block blue light emissions and to limit your device use after the sun goes down.

Supplements

Supplements are an important part of anyone's diet, especially when your body is adjusting to working in ketosis or entering a fast. I usually take supplements when I eat for better absorption.

If you're eating correctly, you'll be getting most of these nutrients on your own, but it is still a good idea to know where you can do better. You can even focus on your vitamin health naturally without purchasing anything in pillform.

For example, two of the best sources of magnesium and potassium are meat and green vegetables. But the way we prepare both drains them of their nutrients. In meat, the drippings contain most of the magnesium and potassium. Use the drippings to make a sauce to capture these nutrients. You have probably noticed that when you boil vegetables, the water turns green. Again, this is where the magnesium and potassium end up. Drink some of this or steam the vegetable to preserve the nutrients in the vegetables.

The list of supplements you can take is endless, but here are the ones I believe are critical, listed in order of importance.

Here are the vitamins and minerals you need to make sure you are taking:

Supplements

Electrolyte Replenisher

MAGSRT – *This is number two, right after a general electrolyte replenisher. This is another electrolyte that needs replenishing.*

GNH – *This is your probiotic/prebiotic and is healing the gut.*

Vitamin C / Vitamin D3 – *Make sure to take a slow-release version of these products, which are taken together for absorption.*

Kelp pills – *A natural source of iodine, which supports your thyroid function.*

Krill fish oil – *The best source of omega-3's.*

Spirulina (blue-green algae) – *High in proteins and vitamins, as well as potentially an anti-inflammatory.*

Zymphlomed, Numeric *(or any comparable product) – These are herbs that reduce and balance out inflammation.*

Multi-vitamin – *A general multi is optional if you're eating enough vegetables. Make sure it doesn't have sugar in it!*

Green powder – *This is your alternative to a pre-biotic.*

Daily multi or organ powder
Calcium, magnesium, and zinc
Potassium
L-carnitine
BCAA
Salt
Kelp – Iodine supplement
Blue-Green Algae
Probiotic and Prebiotic

Inflammation reductions supplements:

* *Rosemary*
* *Turmeric*
* *Ginger*
* *Holy Basil*
* *Organic Green Tea*
* *Hu Zhang*
* *Chinese goldthread*
* *Barberry*
* *Organic oregano*
* *Chinese skullcap*
* *Ground cinnamon*

CHAPTER 5: WOMEN'S HORMONES AND KETOSIS

THE COMPLEXITY WITH WOMEN, HORMONES, AND WEIGHT LOSS

Before beginning this chapter, go watch this introduction to rebalancing women's hormones:

https://www.metabolicrenewal.com/p/aff/video?ht=2&pmadid=1152765

Women's bodies are more complex than men's when it comes to weight loss. Women have different hormones, different metabolisms, and a different relationship with body stress. This chapter will explore how women's specific hormones interact with and impact weight loss, including why women are able to lose weight in certain portions of the month but not others.

Finally, we will wrap up with a section focused on cultivating a relaxed mindset that will be useful for anyone's health journey, not just women's.

All About the Hormones

Women's ability to lose weight is not as straightforward as men's. Why? At this point in the book I am sure the answer will no longer surprise you: it's all about the hormones.

Every month, hormones fluctuate for women who are post-puberty but pre-menopausal because of their menstrual cycle. Many women have probably noticed they bloat and gain weight when they are on their period. If you track your weight regularly, you might have noticed that there are some weeks that weight is more stubborn about coming off. That isn't because you aren't being disciplined about your keto diet or exercise. That is fundamentally a matter of what is happening hormonally in your body.

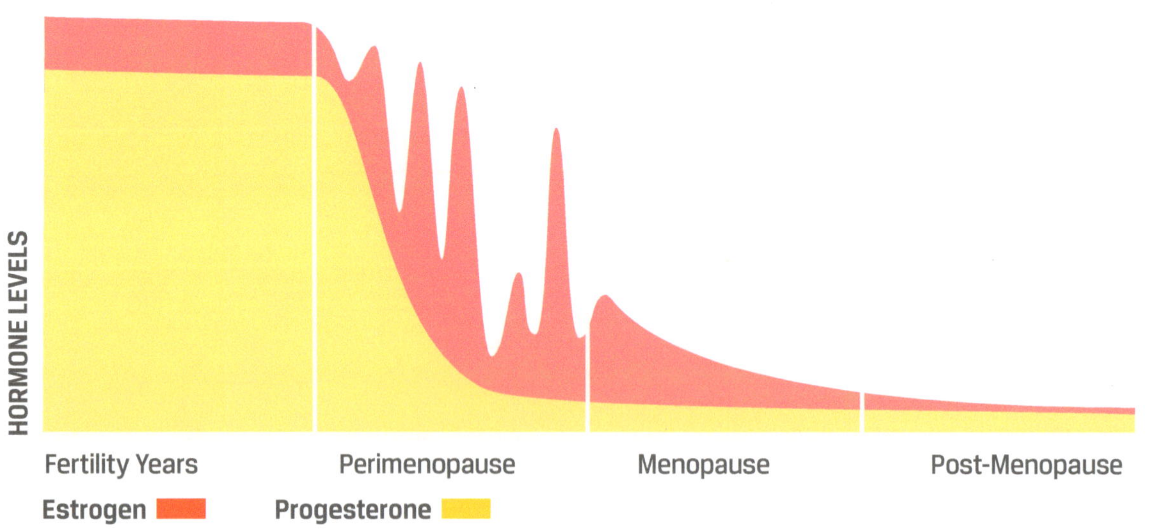

FIG 5.1 ***Female Hormonal Lifecycle***

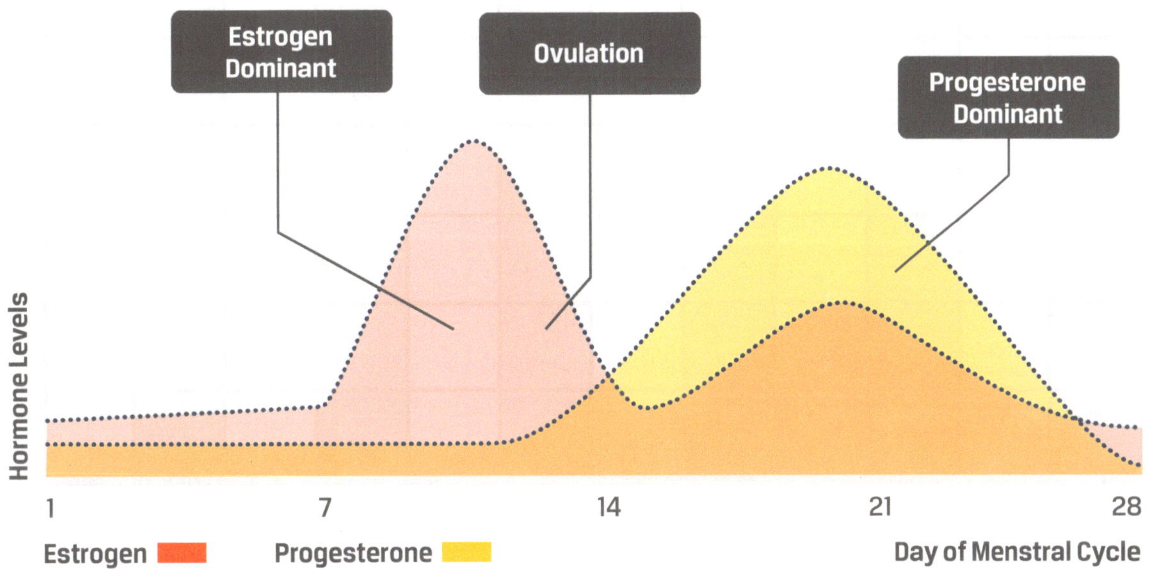

FIG 5.2 ***Menstral Cycle Hormone Levels***

Based on the work of Dr. Jade Teta, women need to make adjustments to their eating and workout plans depending on their natural female hormonal rhythms.

Just look at the dramatic changes to female hormones that happen throughout life *[FIG 5.1]*.

Or what happens each and every month during the menstrual cycle *[FIG 5.2]*.

Throughout women's lives, their estrogen and progesterone hormones fluctuate wildly, and these aren't the only two hormones at play. Another key biological difference between men and women is that the female metabolism is much more sensitive to cortisol.

One study showed that 75% of doctor visits for women are stress-related. When you are stressed, your body releases the hormone cortisol, which impairs thyroid function and slows down your metabolism. Cortisol increases hunger and also fat accumulation around the belly.

So, what do you do?

The answer also lies in the hormones *[FIG 5.3]*.

Most women think that estrogen and progesterone are the most important hormones when it comes to fat storage or burning. In fact, *insulin, cortisol, thyroid, and adrenals* are most important when it comes to fat loss.

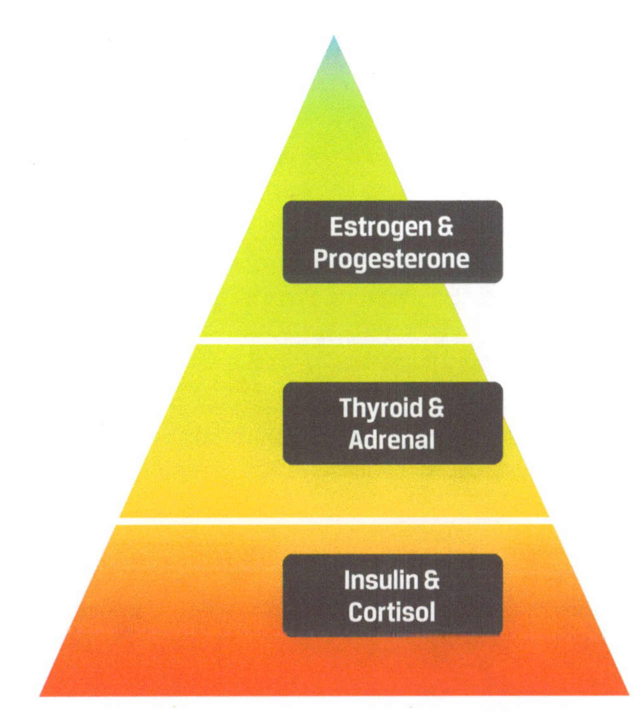

FIG 5.3 ***Hormones and Fat Storage***

Insulin: The Fat Storer

In the hierarchy of hormonal influencers for fat loss, insulin still reigns as queen. This hormone, relative to the others, is most strongly influenced by carbohydrate intake and overconsumption of food, both of which cause a detrimental increase in blood sugar. Women will become more or less insulin-sensitive as their levels of estrogen and progesterone rise and fall.

Cortisol: The Stress Hormone

Cortisol, secreted from the adrenal glands, has a split personality in the body. In other words, it is not all bad or all good. Acute stressors on the body tend to cause a short-term increase of this hormone. It gets the body primed to either fight or flee from the stress. This served us well in Paleolithic times when we were not at the top of the food chain.

Thyroid: The Metabolic Manager

Thyroid hormone, secreted from the thyroid gland, helps to manage the body's metabolic processes, including your fat-burning potential. It is like the thermostat on your metabolism. This hormone is also keenly sensitive to your daily lifestyle choices, including sleep (how long and how deep), nutrition (types and amounts), stress (acute or chronic), and exercise (longer moderate intensity or shorter high intensity.)

The Adrenals: The Metabolic Gas Pedal

Epinephrine and norepinephrine, referred to as catecholamines, along with cortisol, get secreted by the adrenal glands any time you are stressed. This happens especially when you exercise. The great thing about the catecholamines is that they tell the body to get ready to start burning fat.

Estrogen & Progesterone

[Reference FIG 5.2] Estrogen causes fat storage around the hips, butt, breasts, and thighs that gives you that hourglass figure. Progesterone normally works with estrogen to keep fat from accumulating in the center of the body.

When estrogen gets too high and starts to dominate, you will notice a thicker layer of fat around the butt, thighs, and hips. The excess estrogen needs to be removed from the body to get back to balance between estrogen and progesterone.

What do you do? **Fiber** is the key to balancing these hormones. Eat plenty of it, and your issues will be mitigated. Also, moving to organic, non-GMO vegetables will lower your intake of mimicking estrogens in food. Same is true of your meat; you are what your animals eat. Look to buy grass-fed beef and pastured chicken to avoid ingesting GMO grain-fed meat.

If you have ingested a high amount of mimicking estrogens, there is an easy answer. Sweating will help purge those bad boys.

HIGH FIBER KETO FOOD:

* Chia seed, flaxseed, psylium: add to a shake or smoothie
* Broccoli
* Cauliflower
* Red cabbage
* Mushrooms
* Blackberries and raspberries: limit to one cup to stay in ketosis

Managing Your Hormones

As you can see in the graph of hormone fluctuations for women during the month, the month has two distinct phases wherein in estrogen predominates and then progesterone predominates. This first phase is called the follicular phase, while the second is known as the luteal phase.

The kinds of workouts and nutritional plans you pursue will depend on which part of the menstrual cycle you are in.

What to do:

Day 1 to 14 is the follicular phase (EMEM) wherein you eat more and exercise more.

* When estrogen is high, you can tolerate more food and exercise because you are insulin-sensitive. Your muscle will uptake food to build muscle, and your body will lean toward fat loss in calorie deficit.
* Work out 5 days a week (3-15-minute HIIT workouts); (see video; do burn-out & weights)
* Add a couple cardio sessions or yoga sessions
* Walk for 1 to 2 hours per day (5,000 to 10,000 steps; more important than exercise)
* 2 meals with protein, veggies, and starches
* 1 meal with protein and veggies
* Decrease stress with 3 to 5 steam sauna sessions or hot baths; important to sweat and be relaxed

HORMONES:

"Most women think that estrogen and progesterone are the most important hormones when it comes to fat storage or burning. In fact, insulin, cortisol, thyroid, and adrenals are most important when it comes to fat loss."

Day 15 to 28 is luteal phase (ELEL) where you eat less and exercise less.

* When progesterone is high, you need to eat less because the body is more insulin-resistant and prone to storing fat from excess calories. Also, stick to the 3 workouts during these 2 weeks.
* Less exercise (3-15-minute HIIT workouts see video; skip burnout videos)
* Walk for 1 to 2 hours per day (5,000 to 10,000 steps; more important than exercise)
* 2 meals with protein and veggies
* 1 meal with starch at end of day or add glucose and fructose to morning shake post-workout
* More protein in second half because of insulin resistance
* Decrease stress with 3 to 5 steam sauna sessions or hot baths; important to sweat and be relaxed

Still Not Losing Weight

Ensuring that weight loss can happen for you during your cycle is tricky but possible. Here are three key factors every woman should follow that will dramatically change the results they get during this time:

Step 1: Change your meals with a hormone-first approach and adjustments based on cycles

* Need fiber to get rid of excess estrogen
* 30 grams minimum to 100 grams as target per day of fiber plus a ton of water to flush excess estrogen
* Drink whey protein shake with fiber for breakfast
* Big salad for lunch
* Small salad for dinner
* Organic foods to avoid: synthetic estrogen in food from GMOs and Roundup

Step 2: Reduce stress.

I understand just telling someone to be less stressed is not helpful, but I am not nagging. We have a scientific purpose here: cortisol reduction.

* First: stop beating yourself up. If you aren't losing weight, it isn't because you're not trying or not disciplined. Your body just has a different agenda.
* Rest more and relax vs. more cardo and working out; this is making it worse
* Vacation eating, eat whatever you want and resting; many women come back thinner because cortisol was reduced from the lower stress of letting it all go
* Go out with girlfriends and have a glass of wine vs. working out. Really.
* Do saunas or hot baths with Epsom salts
* Get more sleep, as sleep deprivation raises cortisol production. Take a nap. Sleep in.
* Get a massage or take up meditation

Step 3: More movement:

* Lowers insulin as a result
* Talk a walk at 3 miles/hr—slow
* Walking lowers your stress hormones and cortisol

Step 4: Metabolic workouts for women

* 15 minutes, 3 days a week
* Short, intelligent workouts
* Long workouts send you into hormonal tail spin; too much workout for women causes fat storage vs. loss because of the stress on the body.
* These short workouts will trigger HGH (human growth hormone) to shape the female body. Women produce 93% more HGH when working out than men.
* Study of traditional workout vs. the short workout indicates that short workouts lead to 10x more fat loss
* Anaerobic threshold triggers HGH for women
* Basically HIT peak, rest, peak, rest for 15 minutes:
    - Monday - 15 minutes of HIIT(high intensity interval training)
    - Tuesday - walk for 30 minutes, slow pace
    - Wednesday - 15 minutes of HIIT
    - Thursday - walk for 30 minutes, slow pace
    - Friday - 15 minutes of HIIT
* Results of HIIT vs. long workouts for women were twice the toned muscle and 992% more fat loss after 11-week trial

REST-BASED LIVING RECOMMENDATIONS FOR EVERYONE

Having lower stress isn't just a matter of what kinds of hormones you have. Men can absolutely benefit from relaxation as well. Sometimes we want to stimulate stress hormones, but other times we want to relax the body and lower those hormones so that we aren't permanently in a state of stress. Too much of that and the body is never able to rebuild and rebalance.

In addition to what you are eating and doing exercise-wise, there are several key ways that you can lower cortisol in your body.

* Laughing
* Physical affection
* Sweating (i.e. saunas, hot baths)
* Walking
* Massages
* Meditation
* Sleep

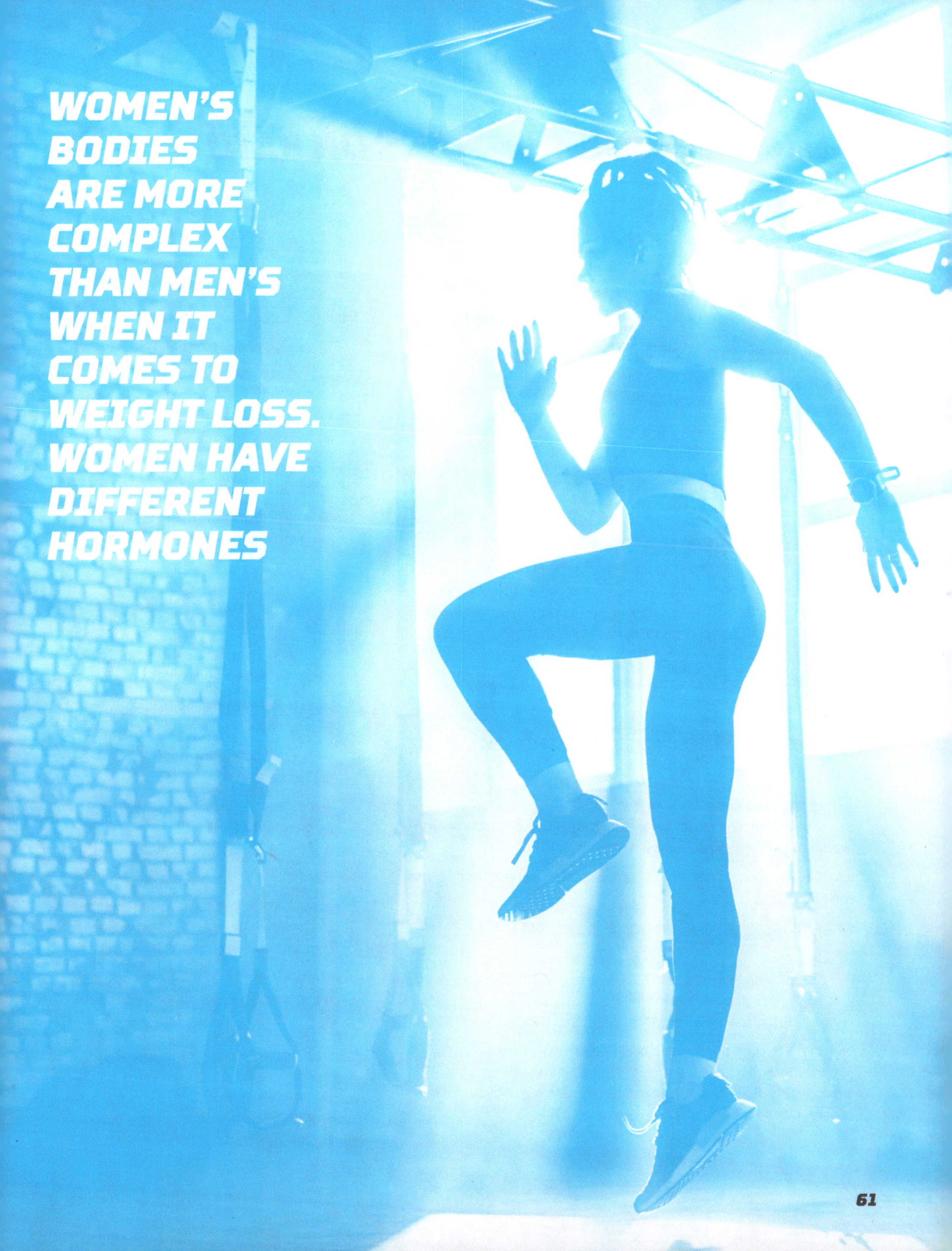

WOMEN'S BODIES ARE MORE COMPLEX THAN MEN'S WHEN IT COMES TO WEIGHT LOSS. WOMEN HAVE DIFFERENT HORMONES

CHAPTER 6: KETO AND BODYBUILDING

BUILDING MUSCLE MASS ON KETO

One of the many myths about keto is that it is impossible to build muscle mass while on a ketogenic diet.

This is patently untrue and unscientific. This chapter describes in detail how to bodybuild on a ketogenic diet. This is an advanced topic, but a personal interest of mine that also showcases how it is possible to tweak keto to fit an athletic lifestyle.

You have been on keto for a while, and it's working. How do you know when to embark on this new program? Once your initial weight loss plateaus, it is time to change things up.

Those last 10 to 15 pounds you want to lose are going to require a different approach than the basic keto or fasting you have been using. The principles are the same. Extend your fast to 18 hours and isolate your eating to a 6-hour period.

On the adjacent page is an example of a macro that will help you accomplish this:

Courtesy of: www.ketosavage.com/keto-macro-calculator/

Building Muscle While in Ketosis

One of the most common myths is that you can't build muscle while in ketosis. Once again, science proves differently.

Here are two studies that show it is absolutely possible to build muscle while in ketosis:

www.jissn.biomedcentral.com/articles/10.1186/1550-2783-11-S1-P40

Study 1:

Half the study participants were fed a high carbohydrate diet (55% carbs, 25% fat, 20 % protein) versus the other half who were fed a ketogenic diet (70% fat, 20% protein, 5% carbs) for 11 weeks.

Twenty-six college-aged, resistance-trained men split between the two groups did a resistance-training program three times per week over 11 weeks. Body fat and lean mass were determined by dual x-ray absorptiometry (DXA) scans.

Results:

* The ketogenic diet group had twice the lean body mass increase of the standard high carbohydrate diet group
* 4.3kgs added vs 2.2kgs lean mass added on average by DXA scans
* Fat loss of 2.2kgs vs. 1.5kgs for the high carbohydrate diet
* More muscle gain and more fat loss for the ketogenic diet

Study 2:

Here is an example of why people say you lose muscle on the ketogenic diet:

* 25 college-aged men were divided up into ketogenic diet vs. traditional western diet
* Important to note that both groups were eating a traditional western diet before
* Weeks 1–10 both groups did resistance training
* Week 11 keto group started eating carbohydrates for 1 week
* Body composition was measured at week 0, 10, and 11
* At week 10, the ketogenic group showed an increase of 2.4% vs. 4.4% of lean muscle mass compared to the traditional western diet
* At week 11, after carb reload, the ketogenic group showed a 4.4% vs. 4.4% increase of lean muscle mass

During the first 10 weeks the muscles, glycogen is depleted, giving the appearance of muscle loss or slower muscle gain. This is because every gram of stored carbohydrate is accompanied by 3 grams of water in glycogen. Once they replenished their glycogen, the overall before and after showed more gain by the ketogenic group.

Higher Protein Intake

You want to have a huge surplus on lifting days.

Macros

- 0.8 to 1 gram of protein per lb. of body weight 18% to 20 % of calories
- 75% of calories from fat
- 2 to 5% calories from carbs

My example at 185 pounds:

* 0.8 to 1 gram of protein per lb. (145 gram) 580 calories 20%
* 76% of calories from fat = 2,204 calories, 244 grams
* 2,900 calories in total
* 4% 116 calories from carbs or 29 grams

Key notes:

* Add in some fasting days in to reduce calories for week to avoid fat gain
  - Train in the morning-fasted state
  - Break your fast with whey protein shake no fat at end of day-fat loss rest of day
  - Protein synthesis stays elevated for 24 hours after workout
* 5% net surplus in calories for the week to build muscle
* Ketones should be between 1 and 2 mmols

Great video to watch:
www.youtu.be/mk9lFY20aWY

Keto Macro Calculator

BODY WEIGHT (LBS)*	180
BODY FAT % (ESTIMATE)	18
BODY FAT WEIGHT (LBS)	32.4
LEAN BODY MASS (LBS)	147.6
LEAN BODY MASS (KGS)	67.09
BMR	1819.14
ACTIVITY MULTIPLIER	AVERAGE 1.50 … EXTRA ACTIVE
TDEE (KCAL)	2728.71
INDUCTION PHASE 30% Reduction	
INDUCTION PHASE CALORIES	1910.10
FAT Grams	169.79
PROTEIN Grams	71.63
CARB Grams	23.88
CARB SURPLUS	IF CARB GRAMS > 10, ADD AMOUNT OVER 10 TO THE DAILY PROTEIN GRAMS
CONFIRMATION PHASE 20% Reduction	
CONSOLIDATION PHASE CALORIES	2182.97
FAT Grams	194.04
PROTEIN Grams	81.86
CARB Grams	27.29
CARB SURPLUS	IF CARB GRAMS > 15, ADD AMOUNT OVER 15 TO THE DAILY PROTEIN GRAMS
MAINTENANCE PHASE 10% Reduction	
MAINTENANCE PHASE CALORIES	2455.84
FAT Grams	204.65
PROTEIN Grams	122.79
CARB Grams	30.70
CARB SURPLUS	IF CARB GRAMS > 20, ADD AMOUNT OVER 20 TO THE DAILY PROTEIN GRAMS
LEAN MASS GAIN	
LEAN MASS GAIN CALORIES	3001.58
FAT Grams	250.13
PROTEIN Grams	150.08
CARB Grams	37.52
CARB SURPLUS	IF CARB GRAMS > 20, ADD AMOUNT OVER 20 TO THE DAILY PROTEIN GRAMS
ACCELERATED FAT LOSS	
FAT LOSS CALORIES	2182.97
FAT Grams	181.91
PROTEIN Grams	109.15
CARB Grams	27.29
CARB SURPLUS	IF CARB GRAMS > [illegible], ADD AMOUNT OVER 20 TO THE DAILY PROTEIN GRAMS

Target Ketogenic Diet (TKD)

This is a specialized diet used by keto bodybuilders. The key lies in post-workout carbs (yes, I said carbs).

Post-workout, perhaps 30 to 60 minutes, the muscles, cells are extra insulin-sensitive. Work out at the end of your fasting period. This will refill your glycogen very quickly and assist with muscle growth.

Study: link.springer.com/article/10.1007%2Fs00421-009-1289-x

* Eat a protein shake with carbs within the first hour of your workout being complete
    - 25 to 30 grams of glucose from dextrose—fast absorbing
    - 15 grams fructose from berries—different absorption pathway from glucose
    - 30 to 50 grams of lean protein from whey protein isolate
    - 2 to 4 grams of omega 3s
    - 1/4 tsp salt is needed to transport the glucose to the cell
    - Coffee
    - No fat!
* Wait 1 hour after work out to eat carbs

You will be back in ketosis by lunch time if you work out in the morning.

Breaking your fast in the manner described above is especially important. I was shocked at the results once I began breaking my fast this way, especially the protein shake with a banana, a fruit I had previously totally avoided. I tested my blood after drinking one of these, and I still had ketones in my blood. This happens because dextrose in the banana shake spikes your insulin, which then shovels the lean protein into muscle cells and re-ups your glycogen.

Good videos: www.youtube.com/watch?v=8SWd5Ra_sRU

Cyclical Ketogenic Diet (CKD)

To do a CKD diet, do your normal ketogenic diet for 5 to 8 days. Then, have one day with carb load to replenish glycogen: 150 grams of carbs. Then, go back to your ketogenic diet.

Work-out plan

To keto bodybuild, you have to work out in a fasted state. This will help your body produce more HGH.

Change the workout up every two weeks to keep seeing results.

Start with your one rep max. Then input the numbers.

www.bodybuilding.com/fun/other7.htm

For two weeks do the following then move on to the next:

* 10 reps at 65-70% of one rep max
* 8 at 75-80% of one rep max
* 6 at 85% of one rep max
* 4 AT 90-95% of one rep max
* 3-4 for sets of one rep max
* All of the support movements should have 8-12 reps

Here is an example if you bench pressed 245 lbs for 8 reps in three sets *[FIG 6.1]*.

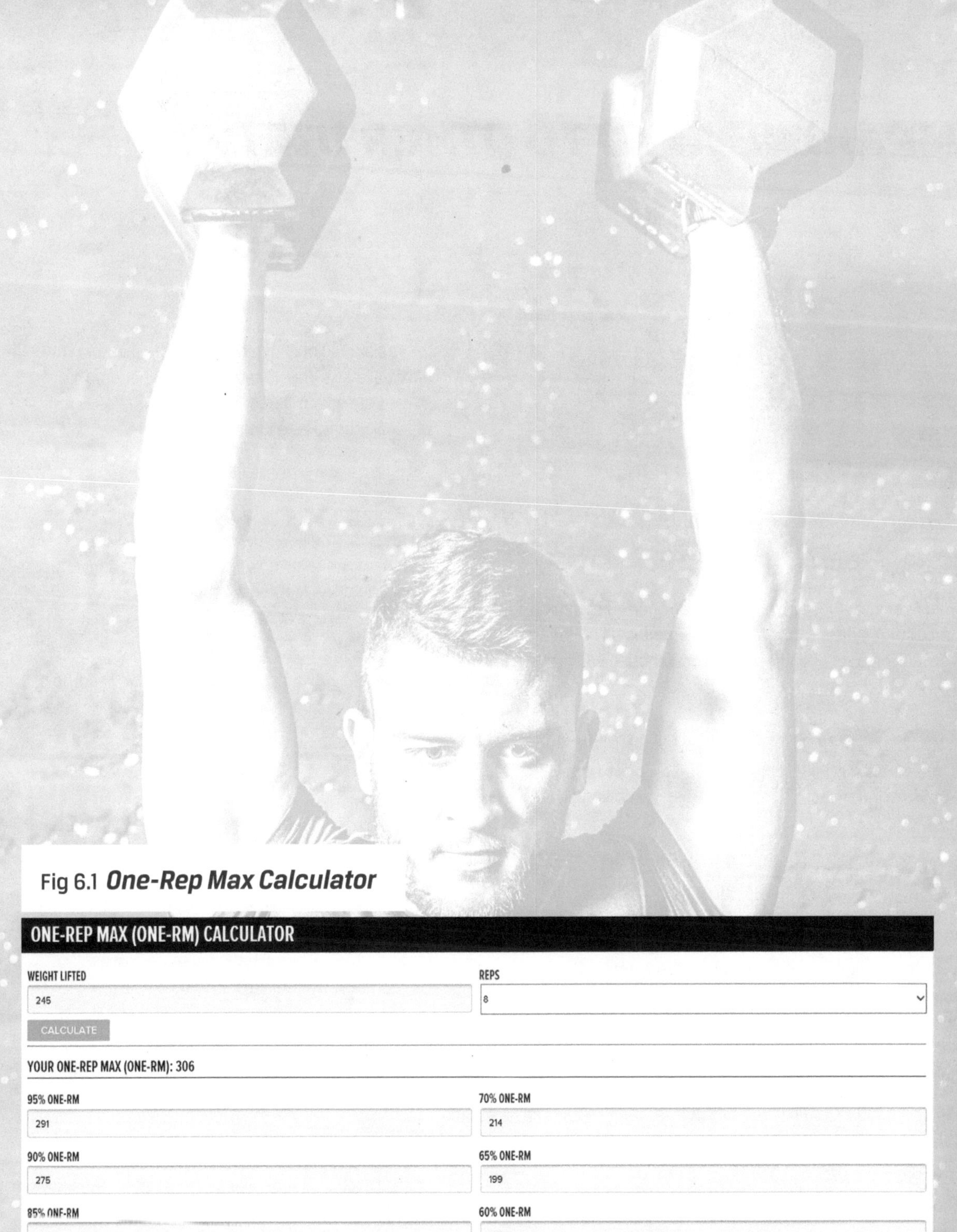

Fig 6.1 ***One-Rep Max Calculator***

ONE-REP MAX (ONE-RM) CALCULATOR

WEIGHT LIFTED	REPS
245	8

CALCULATE

YOUR ONE-REP MAX (ONE-RM): 306

95% ONE-RM	291	70% ONE-RM	214
90% ONE-RM	275	65% ONE-RM	199
85% ONE-RM	260	60% ONE-RM	184
80% ONE-RM	245	55% ONE-RM	168
75% ONE-RM	230	50% ONE-RM	153

COMPARING KETO TO OTHER DIETS

One of the best ways to understand the ketogenic diet is to understand what it is not. Because popular understanding of keto is so limited, it often gets confused for a range of other diets—or just outright misunderstood.

To help dispel some of these myths, I have created a list below of other diets. Some of these diets influenced keto, working as a precursor to what we know now. Other diets can be used in conjunction with keto to target a specific result.

The Carnivore Diet

The carnivore diet is all about removing a ton of foods from your diet that might be causing inflammation. You will consume no veggies or spices, just meat.

PROTOCOL

* ACV first thing in morning
* No bulletproof coffee—black coffee only
* Work out first thing in the morning in a fasted state

Breakfast: Lean meat for first meal such as chicken or salmon (uses fat from stored body fat)

Lunch: Higher fat like ground beef or turkey

Dinner: High fat meat like a rib eye steak (mix of meats is good; like surf and turf to add magnesium to meal)

* Fast two days a week 20 to 24 hours
* Separate days, not back to back
* Work out M, W, F
* Cardio on Monday
* Tuesday and Saturday doing 30 minutes of cardio

You should only use the carnivore diet for two weeks at a time to reduce inflammation. Then go back to a keto diet with vegetables. This is not designed to be a long-term diet.

Paleo

Paleo is what we used to eat a thousand years ago. Its core principle is that we should eat what our bodies evolved to eat (without taking into account the last twelve thousand years). It is quite the rage right now.

In practice, paleo is a moderately low carb diet wherein you consume 50–100 grams of carbs a day. Some people can be in ketosis at this level. Another more minor difference is that there are some vegetables on the paleo diet that aren't allowed on a keto diet.

From a maintenance level, paleo is probably a great diet. You moderate your carbs. You're not falling back into insulin resistance.

It is essentially like eating keto because you're getting enough fiber that the carbs aren't absorbing. Fiber doesn't have the glucose response that causes an insulin spike.

There isn't science to back that we were eating this way in the Paleo period. It is the best alternative to the keto diet, but it won't have the same effects on healing/weight loss.

SAD (Standard American Diet)

The standard American diet includes 300–500 grams of carbs. The worst of all, high carb with high fat. This causes 95% of the fat to be stored directly and never burned because of all the carbs.

South Beach

This diet was uber popular in the late 1990s/2000s. It is the next evolution of the SAD diet. It is low carb and also low fat. People did lose weight on it, because they were essentially starving.

On South Beach, you're not accessing stored fat. Even if you lose a ton of weight due to starving, this kind of calorie-restricted diet leads to shutting down your metabolism.

South Beach became very commercialized, with a lot of products you could buy. But then South Beach bars had sugar and other carbs, etc. They were not following their own advice. In general, South Beach doesn't work for people.

(Just a sidenote: that's why you see keto exploding, because it works.)

Atkins

Atkins was the beginning of examining American myths about "healthy" eating. Just to note, the Atkins diet is old but it has been updated in the last few years. Check out *The New Atkins for a New You* by Dr. Weissman.

This is a very low carb diet, mostly made up of vegetables. All carbs were treated equal.

The creator had a basic idea that ketosis was happening, but didn't have the blood meters or anything to get real data on it. He was helping people with heart disease, which eventually led him to target carbs. But the science was weak. The first clinical trials were run at Duke. This is the beginnings of the keto diet.

APPENDIX A: RECIPES

BREAKFAST

2 eggs w/ 2 Strips of Bacon

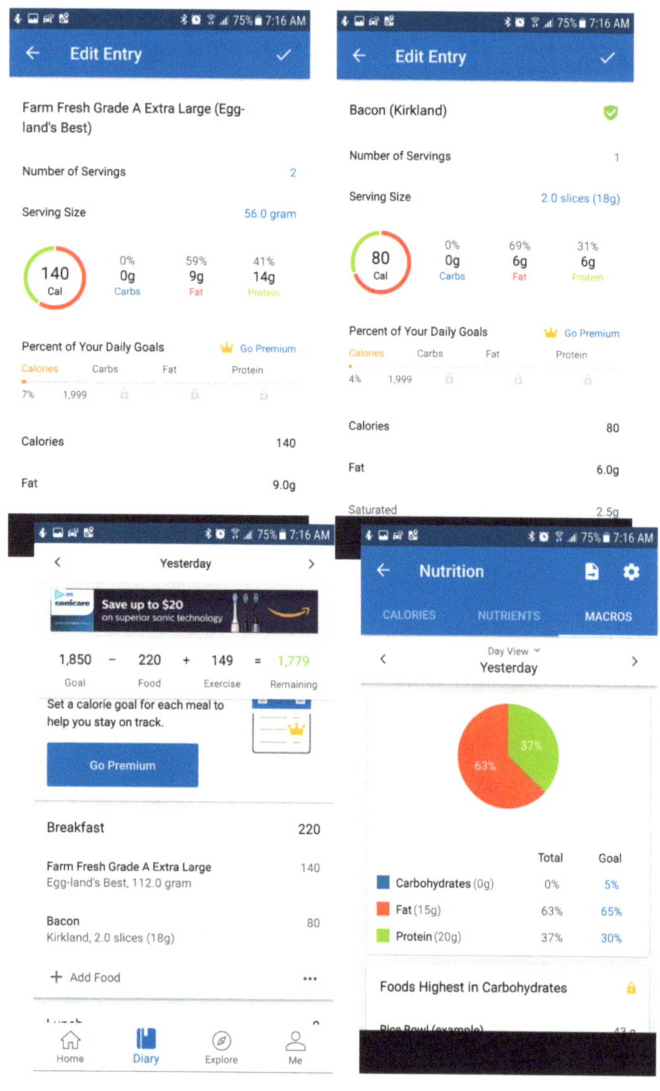

FIG A.1 ***Examples of How to Calculate Macros Using MyFitnessPal-Eggs / Bacon***

2 eggs w/ 2 links of Sausage

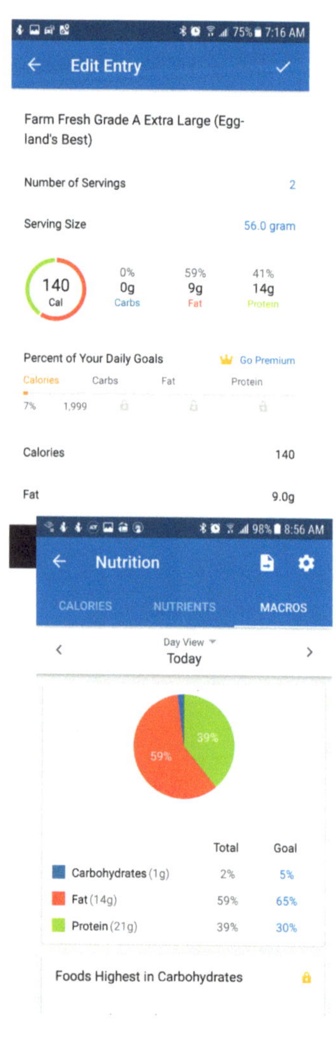

FIG A.2 ***Eggs / Sausage***

Breakfast Casserole

- _ 1 lb. ground beef (80/20)
- _ 12 large eggs
- _ 4 oz. cheddar cheese
- _ ¼ cup heavy cream
- _ 5 cups fresh spinach
- _ 1 tsp pink salt
- _ ½ tsp black pepper

* Heat oven to 350
* Cook ground beef on stove then add spinach to pan for a few minutes
* Mix eggs with heavy cream and salt and pepper
* Put ground beef with spinach in a casserole pan and pour egg mixture over
* Bake 30-40 minutes

Bacon 'N' Cheese Egg Bake

* 12 large eggs
* 2 cups sour cream
* 1.5 cup heavy cream
* 1 tsp sea salt
* ½ tsp ground black pepper
* 4 cups crumbled bacon
* 2 cups shredded Mexican cheese

Cook at 350 for 30 minutes

Protein Shake

- recipe/ whey protein isolate/ grass-fed beef DYMATIZ ISO100 WHEY PROTEIN - CHOCOLATE/PB

Increase fat by adding macadamia nut milk; heavy whipping cream, too. Add a handful of berries in there, and a little bit of salt.

LUNCH

Lunch is oftentimes my first meal of the day. I usually keep my lunch simple.

A key to eating a ketogenic diet is reducing the number of decisions you make in a day. One of the ways I increase efficiency and reduce decision-making is: eating the same thing for lunch and dinner. I make extra servings of my dinner and then pack it up the next day for my lunch. If you need a little more variety, several more options follow.

Last Night's Left-overs

Panino by Fiorucci

Hard Salami wrapped mozzarella cheese

* 300 Calories
* 25 grams of fat
* 2 grams of carbs
* 17 grams of protein

Stuffed Avocado

1 cup of spinach

Handful of sliced red onion

Half an avocado

Scoop of tuna salad, egg salad, or chicken salad

Fried Egg Salad

1 or 2 cups spinach

4 fried eggs with a runny yolk

Garnish with shredded cheese and avocado to taste

Tuna boats

Make a nest of romaine lettuce leaves and put a scoop of tuna salad on them.

Garnish with cheddar cheese

Lunch On the Go Options

* Chicken caesar salad with no croutons
* Cobb salad with no corn or beans

SNACKS

People often ask me what the best snack is while you're eating keto. My honest answer: none. Remember, every time you eat, you're going to experience an insulin spike. There is no need to "keep your metabolism running." It runs fine on its own, especially if you're in fat-burning mode.

If you do need to snack, I have a few options for you. Nuts are a classic, but not nearly as good as meat and cheese. Just try to eat four Babybel cheese wheels. That's only 600 calories in total, but good luck. Another great option is a can of tuna. I keep cans of tuna in my office and a jar of mayo in the fridge. In a pinch, I can mix them together to create an ad hoc tuna salad.

The amount of fat in items like Babybel cheese or tuna salad triggers that leptin so fast, they easily satisfy your hunger cravings.

Roasted Macadamia Nuts

A handful of around 30 nuts will fill you up and is a great ketogenic food

* 200 kCals
* 4 grams of carbs
* 21 grams of fat
* 2 grams of protein

Prosciutto and Provolone Cheese

Pack by Primo Taglio

* 220 Calories
* 0 grams of carbs
* 15 grams of fat
* 23 grams of protein

Mini Babybel Cheese

The red ones - full fat

* 70 calories
* 0 grams of carbs
* 6 fat
* 5 protein

DINNER

Pork Chops

- ghee 1-2 Tbsp based on chops size
- garlic

SAUCE

- one container of cream cheese
- one cup of broth
- Italian seasoning
- salt and pepper
- ¼ cup of parmesan cheese

BBQ Chicken Lettuce Wraps

- 3 lbs chicken breast
- Low sugar BBQ sauce
- 1 red onion
- Bake chicken with BBQ sauce and red onion 50-60 minutes, 400 degrees (or Crockpot)
- Shred for serving on iceberg lettuce

New York Fat Head Pizza

CRUST:

Melt

* 1 cup mozzarella
* 2 Tbsp of ricotta

Then add

* ½ tsp baking powder
* ½ cup almond flower
* 1 egg

Stir

Season with

* ½ tsp green pesto
* Garlic powder

Put on parchment paper and poke holes in it. Bake at 400 for ten minutes

TOPPINGS:

* Pepperoni on bottom
* Then bacon
* Then mozzarella
* Roast tomato sauce
* Then more mozzarella
* Two scoops of ricotta

Nutritional Information

* 840 Kcals
* Fat 69 grams
* Protein 51 grams
* Carbs 6 grams

Chicken Crust Pizza

* 5 oz canned chicken breast
* Drain it and dry in the oven at 400 for about 5-10 minutes
* Then add ¼ cup grated parmesan cheese and melt mixture in microwave
* Then add on egg to mixture
* Spread out on baking sheet with parchment paper on bottom, use a second piece on top to roll it out thin
* Bake for 10 minutes
* Add basil pesto made with olive oil—check ingredients; many pestos are made with bad oils
* Add pepperoni & ground beef
* Drizzle pizza with olive oil to get fat content up
* Use goat cheese

Egg Roll Bowl

INGREDIENTS:

* 4 ½ oz ground pork
* 1 cup shredded cabbage (cole slaw mix)
* 1 tsp Sriracha
* 5 drops liquid Stevia
* Splash rice wine vinegar
* ½-1 tsp sesame oil
* Optional: 1 large egg

1. Heat a large skillet to medium high heat and add in the ground pork. Break apart into crumbles using a wooden spoon and allow to cook through.
2. Once fully cooked through, add in the cabbage and stir to combine.
3. Add in the Sriracha, stevia, and rice wine vinegar and stir to combine.
4. Transfer to a bowl and drizzle with sesame oil.
5. If adding an egg, break into the skillet before transferring the mixture to bowl and stir to combine. Allow egg to cook through to your liking.

Keto hamburger patties with creamy tomato sauce and fried cabbage

Ketogenic low carb

Per serving

Net carbs: 4 % (10 g)

Fiber: 5 g

Fat: 77 % (78 g)

Protein: 19 % (43 g)

kcal: 924

Store Bought Pizza

Realgood Pizza Company has the perfect keto- and diabetic-friendly personal pizza for any occassion!

Keto Gravy

Anytime you cook meat, onions, and mushrooms in your crock pot, make sure you retain the drippings at the bottom of the pot. This is your keto gravy.

I like to save mine and use it as a topping for cauliflower rice, which is available in single-serve microwave packages from most grocery stores.

DESSERT

Keto Peanut Butter & Chocolate Chip Ice Cream

* 2 cups heavy whipping cream
* ¼ cup powered Stevia or Sugar in the Raw
* 2 Tbsp of peanut butter powders

CHOCOLATE AND PEANUT BUTTER CUPS

* ½ cup coconut oil
* ½ cup peanut butter
* 4 Tbsp of powdered cooking cocoa
* 6 Tbsp of Stevia
* 1 tsp of vanilla extract

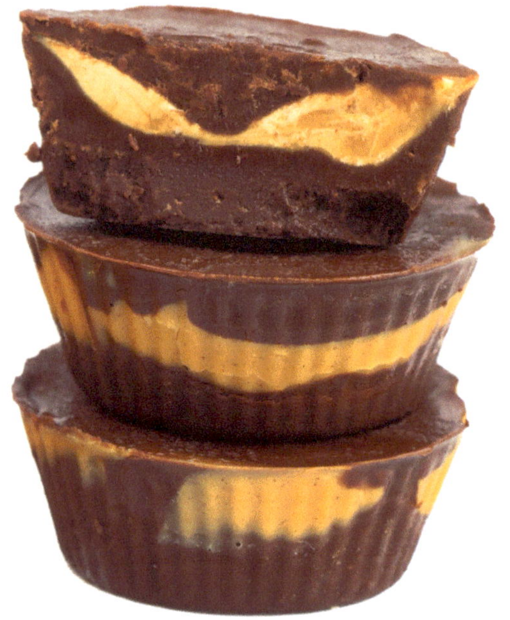

Keto Chocolate Bars

* 1 cup almond butter
* 5 Tbsp of coconut oil
* ¼ tsp of salt
* ¼ tsp of cinnamon
* 5 scoops of vanilla protein powder
* ½ tsp of Swerve
* Some coco snaps

Macadamia Nut Fat Bobs

* 12 Tbsp coconut oil
* 1 ½ oz macadamia nuts
* 1 scoop protein powder
* Sprinkle pink salt

Chocolate Chip Cookie Dough

* 1 ¼ cup almond flour unblanched
* ⅓ cup stevia blend (Swerve brand)
* ⅓ cup almond butter
* ⅓ cup sugar-free syrup
* 1 scoop vanilla whey protein powder
* ½ cup sugar free chocolate chips
* ¼ tsp salt

SWAP OUT

Ice Cream

Killer Whey Ice cream has 2 net carbs

Halo Top also has some good options at about 8 net carbs per serving.

Alcohol

BEER

There are many low carb beers out now:

* Bud Select 55 has 55 calories and 1.9 carbs per 12 oz.
* Amstel Xlight - 2 carbs per 12 oz.
* Michelob Ultra - 2.6 carbs per 12 oz. (my favorite)
* Miller Lite - 3.2 carbs per 12 oz.
* Corona Premier - 2 carb per 12 oz. (make sure it is Premier and not Light, which has 5 carbs)
* Stay away from Coors Light: it has 5 carbs, and Bud Light has 6.6 carbs.

WINE

Wine doesn't have as many carbs in it as you would think. A normal glass of red or white wine will have 2-3 carbs per glass. Champagne, surprisingly, is even lower: around 1 gram per glass.

I recently found a company that will ship cases of wine or Champagne to your house that they test to be low in sugar and a bunch of other items.

Dry Farm

Below is a statement from Dry Farm Wines:

"We consider sugar and alcohol to be toxins. Because we care about what we consume, we apply a rigorous testing protocol to every wine, including independent lab testing for sugar, alcohol, and sulfur levels. We only source wines that meet the following purity standards:

* Statistically Sugar Free. Every wine is fermented completely dry, with less than 0.15 grams per 5oz glass. This includes rosé, sparkling, and white wine.
* Lower Alcohol. With the national alcohol average nearing 15%, our wines never surpass 12.5% alc/vol, with some as low as 7%.
* Lower Sulfites. Our wines average a very low 39 parts per million. In the US, by law sulfites are allowed in amounts up to 350 parts per million (ppm) in wine.
* No Additives. While commercial wine companies may use up to 70+ FDA-approved additives, including thickeners and dyes, to create a shelf-stable product.
* All Native Yeast. Our pure Natural Wines are only fermented with wild, native yeast growing naturally on grapes. Commercial wines are fermented with GMO lab-cultured yeasts."

SPIRITS

Most pure spirits have no carbs in them. Vodka, whiskey, tequila, and rum are all okay. It's usually the mixer that adds all the sugar.

I enjoy a mixed drink often with 2 oz. of liquor mixed with a flavored carbonated water. No carbs. Zevia makes my favorite mixers and sodas with stevia vs. some of the other sweeteners.

There are even low-carb margarita mixes now.

Sauces

You need to be very careful with sauces, as most of them are loaded with sugar. If you carefully search the aisle, you will find lower sugar versions of the products that will allow you to enjoy your sauces without messing up your macros and kicking you out of ketosis.

KETCHUP

Regular Heinz has 8 grams of carbs per Tbsp.
Heinz No Sugar Added only has 1 gram per Tbsp.

RANCH

Primal Kitchen makes a good one out of avocado oil, or you can make your own.

Ranch dry mix

* 2 tsp ground black pepper
* ¾ cup dried parsley flakes
* ⅓ cup garlic powder
* ⅓ cup onion powder
* 2 Tbsp salt
* 1 Tbsp dried dill

The dressing

* 2 Tbsp of the dry ranch mix
* ¾ cup mayonnaise
* ¾ cup sour cream
* ¾ cup heavy whipping cream
* ½ tsp lemon juice

BBQ SAUCE

Lillie's Q has zero-sugar BBQ sauces

MAYONNAISE

You want to find one not made from seed oil (corn, HFCS, or others).
Look for ones made from avocado, coconut, or olive oil.

Primal Kitchen has a few good keto-friendly offerings::

COFFEE CREAMER

Their creamer is made from the highest-quality blend of grass-fed butter, MCT oil, and grass-fed whey protein. The taste is reminiscent of classic half-and-half creamer and contains zero grams of sugar. Whether you drink decaf from a pour-over, crave cold-brew, or have a morning matcha habit, their creamer effortlessly mixes into your beverage of choice—regardless of whether it's hot or cold.

SODA AND FLAVORED WATERS

Zevia make a whole product offering with Stevia as the sweetener

Oils

Vegetable oils have been marketed as "heart healthy" over the last few decades as they were lower in saturated fat. We now know that these products are much worse for us than what we used to cook with.

Bad oils: anything made from a seed, because they have high levels of omega-6 fatty acids and are now classified as trans-fats.

AVOID VEGETABLE OILS:

* Soy
* Canola
* Corn
* Cotton
* Sunflower
* Safflower

GOOD OIL:

* Coconut oil
* Olive oil
* Avocado oil
* Palm oil
* Ghee
* Almond oil
* Sesame oil
* Fish oil
* Lard
* Peanut oil

(I recommend avoiding the peanut oil due to the lectins; see chapter on the gut.)

You can get spray coconut and olive oil now in a can for cooking.

Chips and Crackers

Most chips are made of potatoes or corn, which rules them out. If you are missing chip for dips, try using pork rinds. Pork rinds are also an excellent substitute for breading on food; just crush them up and roll the meat in egg then in the pork rinds.

There are several cracker choices out there:

CRACKERS

Refer to website for current list of recommended vendors:
www.theketocoach.com

Meat

Not all meat is created equal. Your meat is what it eats, so if the cows are feed GMO corn and soy, you will get the GMOs in your meat. The same is true with chicken and eggs; what they are fed matters.

Refer to website for current list of recommended vendors:
www.theketocoach.com

Fruit/Miscellaneous

* Berries (blueberries, strawberries, raspberries) can be enjoyed occasionally in small amounts, as they are the lowest in carbohydrates. Avoid other types of fruit, as most are too high in carbs and can interfere with ketosis.
* Japanese Shirataki noodles
* Pork Rinds (see above; these are great with dip, or as a substitute for bread crumbs, but note they are also high in protein, so limit amounts).

Sweeteners

Avoiding sweetened foods in general will help "reset" the taste buds. However, if there is a desire for something sweet, these are the recommended choices for sweeteners. Note that the powdered forms of most artificial sweeteners usually have maltodextrin, dextrose, or some other sugar added, so liquid products are preferred.

* Stevia—liquid preferred as the powdered usually has maltodextrin in it.
* Erythritol
* Xylitol (keep any food with this sweetener in it away from dogs)
* Splenda—liquid preferred as the powdered usually has maltodextrin in it.
* Lo Han Guo
* Monk Fruit
* Inulin and Chicory Root (Just Like Sugar brand)

My latest favorites are Swerve and liquid Stevia for coffee.

Food Tables

https://www.ketogenic-diet-resource.com/low-carb-food-list.html

Food Item	Calories	Fat (g)	Carbs (g)	Fiber (g)	Net Carbs	Protein (g)
Almond meal (flour), 1 oz.	160	14	6	3	3	6
Coconut butter, 2 Tbsp.	186	18	8	4	4	2
Coconut, dried, unsweetened, 1 oz.	165	15	6	4	2	3
Nuts, almond, roasted, 1 oz.	172	16	5	3	2	6
Nuts, Brazil nut, roasted, 1 oz.	186	19	3	2	1	4
Nuts, cashew, 1 oz.	164	14	10	0	10	8
Nuts, hazelnut, 1 oz.	183	18	5	3	2	4
Nuts, macadamia, roasted, 1 oz.	203	22	4	3	1	2
Nuts, pecan, roasted, 1 oz.	201	21	4	3	1	3
Nuts, walnut, 1 oz.	185	18	4	2	2	4
Seeds, chia, 1 oz.	140	10	12	10	2	4
Seeds, flax, 1 oz.	152	12	8	7	1	6
Seeds, pumpkin, roasted, 1 oz.	148	12	4	1	3	9
Seeds, sesame, 1 oz.	161	14	7	5	2	5
Seeds, sunflower, roasted, 1 oz.	168	15	6	3	3	6

Fig B.1 ***Nuts and Seeds***

Food Item	Calories	Fat (g)	Carbs (g)	Fiber (g)	Net Carbs	Protein (g)
Cheese, Blue, 1 oz.	100	8	1	0	0	6
Cheese, Brie, 1 oz.	95	8	0	0	0	6
Cheese, Cheddar, natural, 1 oz.	114	9	0	0	1	7
Cheese, Cottage, 1-2%, 0.25 cup	41	1	2	0	2	7
Cheese, Cream (block), 2 Tbsp.	101	10	1	0	1	2
Cheese, Mexican blend, 1 oz.	105	9	1	0	1	7
Cheese, Monterey Jack, 1 oz.	106	9	0	0	1	7
Cheese, Mozzarella, part skim, 1 oz.	72	5	1	0	1	7
Cheese, Mozzarella, whole milk, 1 oz.	90	7	1	0	1	6
Cheese, Parmesan, hard, 1 oz.	111	7	1	0	1	10
Cheese, Provolone, 1 oz.	100	8	1	0	1	7
Cheese, Ricotta, whole milk, 0.25 cup	107	8	2	0	2	7
Cheese, Swiss, 1 oz.	108	8	2	0	2	8
Cream, heavy, fluid, 2 Tbsp.	103	11	1	0	1	1
Sour cream (full fat, no fillers—e.g. Daisy brand), 4 Tbsp.	120	10	2	0	2	2
Yogurt, Greek, full fat, 3.5 oz.	95	5	4	0	4	9
Yogurt, Greek, 0% fat, 3 oz.	50	0	3.5	0	3.5	9

Fig B.2 ***Dairy Products***

Food Item	Calories	Fat (g)	Carbs (g)	Fiber (g)	Net Carbs	Protein (g)
Avocado Oil, 1 Tbsp.	124	14	0	0	0	0
Avocado, Haas, 3 oz.	102	9	7	5	2	2
Bacon fat, 1 Tbsp.	116	13	0	0	0	0
Beef tallow, 1 Tbsp.	115	13	0	0	0	0
Butter, 1 Tbsp.	102	12	0	0	0	0
Chicken fat, 1 Tbsp.	115	13	0	0	0	0
Cocoa butter, 1 Tbsp.	120	14	0	0	0	0
Coconut oil, 1 Tbsp.	117	14	0	0	0	0
Cream cheese (block), 2 Tbsp.	101	10	1	0	1	2
Flaxseed oil, 1 Tbsp.	120	14	0	0	0	0
Ghee, 1 Tbsp.	112	13	0	0	0	0
Heavy cream, fluid, 2 Tbsp.	103	11	1	0	1	1
Lard, fresh (non-hydrogenated), 1 Tbsp.	115	13	0	0	0	0
Macadamia oil, 1 Tbsp.	120	14	0	0	0	0
Mayonnaise (full fat), 1 Tbsp.	99	11	1	0	1	0
MCT oil, 1 Tbsp.	100	14	0	0	0	0
Olive oil, 1 Tbsp.	119	14	0	0	0	0
Olives, black, 1 cup	141	13	8	4	4	1
Olives, green, 1 cup	193	20	5	4	1	1
Pork rinds, fried, 0.75 oz.	116	7	0	0	0	13••
Red palm oil, 1 Tbsp.	120	14	0	0	0	0
Salad dressing, creamy full fat (2 carb/serving), 1.5 Tbsp.	130	14	1	0	1	1
Sour cream (full fat, no fillers-e.g. Daisy brand), 4 Tbsp.	120	10	2	0	2	2

·· The protein is inferior in quality. Count the protein grams but limit amounts eaten so as not to displace other more complete protein foods.

Fig B.3 ***Fats and Oils***

Food Item	Calories	Fat (g)	Carbs (g)	Fiber (g)	Net Carbs	Protein (g)
Bacon, cooked, 2 slices	92	9	2	0	2	4
Beef, ground, 80% lean, cooked, 1 oz.	74	5	0	0	0	7
Duck, roasted, skin eaten, 1 oz.	95	8	0	0	0	5
Egg, whole, large, plain, 1 ea.	72	5	0	0	0	6
Lamb, boneless, cooked, 1 oz.	83	6	0	0	0	7
Pork breakfast sausage, (no fillers or sugar, cooked), 1.5 oz.	102	9	0	0	0	7
Pork ribs, roasted, plain, 1 oz.	104	8	0	0	0	8
Pork shoulder, roasted, 1 oz.	82	6	0	0	0	7
Beef, ground, 92% lean, cooked, 1 oz.	45	2	0	0	0	7
Beefsteak, broiled or baked, 1oz.	71	4	0	0	0	8
Beef, chuck, blade roast, cooked, 1 oz.	75	4	0	0	0	9
Chicken breast, roasted or baked, skin not eaten, 1 oz.	46	1	0	0	0	9
Chicken thigh, roasted, no skin, 1.0 oz.	55	3	0	0	0	7
Clams, fresh, baked, 1 oz.	39	2	1	0	1	4
Cottage cheese, 1-2%, 0.25 cup	41	1	2	0	2	7
Crab, king, fresh, steamed, 1.5 oz.	41	0	0	0	0	7.5
Egg whites, raw, large egg, 2 ea.	34	0	0	0	.5	7
Elk steak, roasted, 1 oz.	41	.5	0	0	0	8.5
Fish fillet (flounder, sole, scrod) no breading, baked, 2 oz.	49	1	0	0	0	8.5
Fish, salmon fresh fillet, 1 oz.	39	1	0	0	0	7
Fish, salmon, canned pink, 1 oz.	39	1	0	0	0	7
Ham, deli style, lean, 1 oz.	35	1	1	0	1	5
Ham, smoked, spiral, 1 oz.	53	3	1	0	1	5
Pork chops, lean, cooked, 1 oz.	57	3	0	0	0	7
Pork roast, loin, cooked, 1 oz.	70	4	0	0	0	8
Scallops, baked or broiled, 1 oz.	38	1	1	0	1	6
Shrimp, steamed or boiled, 1 oz.	39	1	0	0	0	8
Tuna, canned, water pack, 1 oz.	33	0	0	0	0	7
Turkey breast, roasted, no skin, 1 oz.	38	0	0	0	0	9
Turkey thigh, roasted, no skin, 1 oz.	52	2	0	0	0	8

Fig B.4 ***Sources of Protein***

Food Item	Calories	Fat (g)	Carbs (g)	Fiber (g)	Net Carbs	Protein (g)
Asparagus, cooked, 1 cup	46	2	6	4	2	5
Beans, tooked (black, kidney, chick peas, lentils) 0.25 cup	55	0	10	3	7	4
Beans, green, cooked, 1 cup	44	.4	10	4	6	2
Beans, green, cooked, 0.5 cup	22	.2	5	2	3	1
Broccoli, cooked, chopped, 0.5 cup	27	0	6	3	3	2
Brussel sprouts, raw, 1 cup	38	0	8	3	5	3
Cabbage, green, raw, shredded, 4 oz.	23	0	5	2	3	1
Carrots, baby, raw, 2 oz.	20	0	6	2	4	0
Cauliflower, cooked, 1 cup	28	0	6	2	4	2
Celery, raw, chopped, 1 cup	36	0	7	4	3	2
Cucumber, raw, sliced, 10oz.	29	0	6	2	4	1
Eggplant, raw, 6 oz.	33	0	8	5	3	1
Garlic, 6 cloves	24	0	6	0	6	0
Kale, raw, chopped, 2 oz.	28	0	6	1	5	2
Lettuce, any green leaf, shredded, 3 cups	24	0	6	3	3	3
Lettuce, iceberg, shredded, 3 cups	24	0	6	3	3	0
Lettuce, Romaine, shredded, 3 cups	24	0	6	3	3	3
Mushrooms, button, raw, 6 oz.	37	1	6	2	4	5
Mushrooms, Portabella, raw, 4oz.	29	0	6	2	4	3
Onion, green, 0.5 cup	16	0	4	1	3	1
Onion, white, raw, 0.5 cup	33	0	7	1	6	1
Pepper, bell, raw, 4 oz.	23	0	5	2	3	0
Potato, white, cooked, 0.5 cup	95	4	13	2	11	1
Rice, white, cooked, 0.25 cup	51	0	11	0	11	1
Shallots, chopped, 2 Tbsp.	14	0	4	0	4	0
Spinach, cooked, from frozen, 5 oz.	57	3	5	3	2	4
Spinach, raw, 6 oz.	38	1	6	4	2	1
Squash, spaghetti, cooked, 1 cup	75	0	10	2	8	1
Squash, summer, cooked, sliced, 1 cup	36	0	8	3	5	2
Swiss chard, chopped coarse, 3 cups	21	0	4	2	2	2
Tomato sauce, 0.5 cup	40	0	8	2	6	2
Tomato, raw, 6 oz.	31	0	7	2	5	1
Turnips, raw, 4 oz.	32	0	7	2	5	1
Chinese water chestnuts, 1 oz.	64	.3	14	2	12	1

Fig B.5 ***Fresh Vegetables***

Food Item	*Carbs (Tbsp)*
Allspice, ground	3.0
Basil, dried	0.9
Black pepper	2.4
Caraway seed	0.8
Cardamom, ground	2.4
Cayenne pepper	1.6
Cinnamon, ground	1.7
Cloves	1.7
Coriander seed	0.6
Cumin, ground	2.1
Curry powder	1.6
Fennel seed	0.7
Garlic powder	5.3
Ginger, ground	3.1
Imitation vanilla extract	0.3
Mace, ground	1.6
Nutmeg	2.0
Onion powder	5.2
Oregano, ground	0.4
Paprika	1.2
Parsley, dried	0.3
Peppermint, fresh	0.1
Poppy seeds	1.2
Poultry seasoning	2.0
Pumpkin pie spice	3.1
Sage, ground	0.4
Spearmint, dried	0.3
Tarragon, ground	2.0
Thyme, ground	1.1
Vanilla extract	1.6
White pepper	3.0

Fig B.6 ***Spices***

APPENDIX C: THE KETO LIBRARY

READ UP

* *Keto Clarity* – By Jimmy Moore
* *Keto Cure* – By Jimmy Moore
* *Cholesterol Clarity* – By Jimmy Moore
* *Why We Get Fat* – By Gary Taubes
* *Good Calories, Bad Calories* – By Gary Taubes
* *The Case Against Sugar* – By Gary Taubes
* *The Complete Guide to Fasting* – By Dr. Jason Fung
* *The Obesity Code* – By Dr. Jason Fung
* *The Diabetes Code* – By Dr. Jason Fung
* *Spring Chicken: Stay Young* – By Bill Gifford
* *The Ketogenic Diet for Athletes* – By Charlotte Campbell
* *The New Atkins for a New You* – By Eric C. Westmand, M.D.
* *Keto Bodybuilding* – By Siim Land
* *Eat Stop Eat* – By Brad Pilon
* *The Plant Paradox* – By Steven R. Gundry

CPSIA information can be obtained
at www.ICGtesting.com
Printed in the USA
BVHW060128170321
602706BV00004B/7